HOLLYWOOD

DISCARDED BY
MEMPHIS PUBLIC LIBRARY

SEXUAL HEALTH

**Questions
you
have
. . . Answers
you
need**

Other Books in This Series From the People's Medical Society

Allergies: Questions You Have . . . Answers You Need

Alzheimer's and Dementia: Questions You Have . . . Answers You Need

Arthritis: Questions You Have . . . Answers You Need

Asthma: Questions You Have . . . Answers You Need

Back Pain: Questions You Have . . . Answers You Need

Blood Pressure: Questions You Have . . . Answers You Need

Cholesterol and Triglycerides: Questions You Have . . . Answers You Need

Depression: Questions You Have . . . Answers You Need

Diabetes: Questions You Have . . . Answers You Need

Hearing Loss: Questions You Have . . . Answers You Need

Menopause: Questions You Have . . . Answers You Need

Prostate: Questions You Have . . . Answers You Need

Stroke: Questions You Have . . . Answers You Need

Vitamins and Minerals: Questions You Have . . . Answers You Need

Your Eyes: Questions You Have . . . Answers You Need

Your Feet: Questions You Have . . . Answers You Need

Your Heart: Questions You Have . . . Answers You Need

SEXUAL HEALTH

Questions you have ... Answers you need

By Michael V. Reitano, M.D.
and Charles Ebel

≡People's Medical Society.

Allentown, Pennsylvania

The People's Medical Society is a nonprofit consumer health organization dedicated to the principles of better, more responsive and less expensive medical care. Organized in 1983, the People's Medical Society puts previously unavailable medical information into the hands of consumers so that they can make informed decisions about their own health care.

Membership in the People's Medical Society is $20 a year and includes a subscription to the *People's Medical Society Newsletter*. For information, write to the People's Medical Society, 462 Walnut Street, Allentown, PA 18102, or call 610-770-1670.

This and other People's Medical Society publications are available for quantity purchase at discount. Contact the People's Medical Society for details.

Many of the designations used by manufacturers and sellers to distinguish their products are claimed as trademarks. Where those designations appear in this book and the People's Medical Society was aware of a trademark claim, the designations have been printed in initial capital letters (e.g., Monistat).

© 1999 by Sexual Health Magazine, Inc.
Printed in the United States of America

All rights reserved. No part of this publication may be reproduced or transmitted in any form or by any means, electronic or mechanical, including photocopy, recording or any information storage and retrieval system, without the written permission of the publisher.

Library of Congress Cataloging-in-Publication Data
Reitano, Michael V.
    Sexual health : questions you have . . . answers you need / by Michael V. Reitano, and Charles Ebel.
      p. cm.
    Includes bibliographical references and index.
    ISBN 1-882606-43-4
    1. Hygiene, Sexual—Miscellanea. 2. Sex—Miscellanea.
3. Health promotion—Miscellanea. 4. Sexually transmitted diseases—Prevention—Miscellanea. I. Ebel, Charles. II. Title.
RA788.R39   1999
613.9'5—dc21   98-44625
                                                     CIP

1 2 3 4 5 6 7 8 9 0
First printing, January 1999

CONTENTS

Introduction 7

Chapter 1 In Search of Sexual Health 9
              Sexual Health and Society 10
              Sex and Health: Reframing the Dialogue 16
              First Impressions of Sexual Health 18
              Understanding Gender and Sexual Orientation 21
              Patterns of Sexual Behavior 23
              Achieving Sexual Health 27

Chapter 2 Sexual Function: Taking Pleasure From Sex 31
              The Mechanics of Arousal 31
              Problems and Concerns for Women 39
                  Anorgasmia 39
                  Pain During Intercourse 43
                  Sex and Aging: Hormone Deficiency 44
              Problems and Concerns for Men 49
                  Anorgasmia 49
                  Erectile Problems 52
                  Sex and Aging: Hormone Deficiency 60
              Problems of Desire 63

Chapter 3 Sexually Transmitted Diseases 67
              Bacterial Sexually Transmitted Diseases 70
                  Chlamydia 70
                  Gonorrhea 72
                  Pelvic Inflammatory Disease 75
                  Syphilis 76
                  Vaginitis 78
              Protozoa: Trichomoniasis 78
              Parasites: Scabies and Pubic Lice 79
              Viral Sexually Transmitted Diseases 81
                  Genital Herpes 81
                  Genital Warts 89

     Hepatitis 93
     HIV/AIDS 95
    Safer Sex 100

Chapter 4 **Other Reproductive and Urinary Tract Disorders** .. 109
    Problems and Concerns for Women 109
     Bacterial Vaginosis 109
     Yeast Infection (Vulvovaginal Candidiasis) 116
     Urinary Tract Infections 122
    Problems and Concerns for Men 125
     Prostatitis 125
     Prostate Cancer 128
     Peyronie's Disease 129
     Epididymitis 130
     Orchitis 131
     Testicular Cancer 132
     Other Testicular Problems 134

Chapter 5 **Contraception and Fertility** 137
    Conception 137
    Contraception 140
     Oral Contraceptives 141
     Intrauterine Devices 143
     Implants and Injectables 144
     Male Condoms 146
     Vaginal Barriers 149
     Natural Methods 152
     Emergency Contraception 154
     Abortion 155
    Infertility Issues 157
     Fertility 157
     Infertility 159

Appendix 165

Informational and Mutual-Aid Groups 167

Glossary 169

Suggested Reading 182

Index 183

INTRODUCTION

Ever since the 1960s, most books about sex have been of the "how to" nature. Starting with Alex Comfort's *The Joy of Sex,* there have been hundreds, maybe thousands, of books teaching us new positions, old positions with a new slant or "better" ways to approach or have sex. Obviously, the success of these "how to" guides demonstrates a public interest, if not a craving, for sexual assistance. And why not? Sex is both fun and pleasurable if it occurs in the proper context, and there is nothing wrong with wanting to find out ways to increase the fun and pleasure.

But there is more to sex than just the act of intercourse. Sex carries baggage. It can create an unwanted pregnancy, spread virulent disease, cause a lifetime of misery and pain if forced upon an unwilling partner and ruin relationships when taken to extremes. In other words, sex can be both physically and psychologically painful if it is not fully understood in a healthful way.

And that's exactly why I asked one of the nation's foremost sexual health educators, Michael V. Reitano, M.D., and sexual health writer and expert Charles Ebel to create this book. After reviewing most of the books on sex and sexuality on the market, I discovered the missing link was an easy-to-read, easy-to-understand guidebook on all aspects of sexual health. I wanted a book that I could give to my 88-year-old mother or my 16-year-old daughter without hesitation. I was looking for a book that explained not only the physical aspects of sex but also the issues (both physical and psychological) that come into play. Of course, the book had to talk about sexually transmitted diseases. Yes, it needed to address masturbation. And obviously, it could not ignore homosexuality. In other words, rather than another "how to" book about sex, I saw the need for a "how about" sexual health book.

Clearly, Michael Reitano and Charles Ebel have met my expectations and far surpassed them. This is a book without a sexual bias, without a hidden sexual agenda. No issues are ignored nor are they treated lightly. And the book is free of that preachy tone that so often fills the pages of sex guides. The authors use their expertise to help you better understand sexuality and its related issues. They also provide the kind of information that will assist you in making healthy sexual decisions throughout your life. In other words, this book is a primer, written in a nurturing way, that you or any family member can use to better understand sexuality.

I am sure you will find this to be one of the most useful books you own. Whether for yourself, your partner, your child, your parents or even a sex education class in school, this is truly a book you can use and share over a lifetime. It treats sensitive issues sensitively but honestly. And it treats all issues of sexuality fairly and openly, leaving nothing in the closet that might cause misunderstanding or miscommunication.

We here at the People's Medical Society are honored and delighted to publish this most useful and important book. And we are confident you will find it to be an invaluable resource.

CHARLES B. INLANDER
President
People's Medical Society

Terms printed in boldface can be found in the glossary, beginning on page 169. Only the first mention of the word in the text will be boldfaced.

We have tried to use male and female pronouns in an egalitarian manner throughout the book. Any imbalance in usage has been in the interest of readability.

1 IN SEARCH OF SEXUAL HEALTH

Q: What does sex mean?

A: The word, clearly, is rich in meanings. Sex, first of all, denotes the way we reproduce our species. It is the act by which a man and a woman conceive a child. By extension, the term "sex" also refers to the classification of species into male and female based on our biological equipment and function.

For human beings, however, sex has a mysterious power beyond reproductive efficiency, and we express sexual attraction in ways that other species don't. In the fullest sense of the word, sex is a giving or sharing of pleasure that goes beyond reproduction, beyond genital-to-genital contact. It can be an expression of love and spiritual union between two people. Or it can be more simply a celebration of physical pleasure—what some would call recreational sex.

Q: Isn't sexual pleasure a pretty broad concept?

A: Absolutely. That's one of the things that's so intriguing about sex. The goal is usually **orgasm**, the contractions and highly pleasurable sensations that often culminate sexual activity. We humans have many ways of attaining this pleasure, some of which have little to do with reproducing the species.

But even orgasm isn't a gold standard. Rather than cataloguing the acts we consider sexual, as journalist Greta Christina writes, we can think of sex as "the conscious, consensual, mutually acknowledged pursuit of shared sexual pleasure"—by whatever means the imagination can devise. This may be broad, but it's probably as good a definition as any.

Q: Does having sex require having a partner?

A: Giving sexual pleasure to oneself, or **masturbation**, is surely an important part of sexual expression, as we discuss in chapters 1 and 2. When we use the term "having sex," however, we mean the pursuit of sexual pleasure with a partner. This partnership can involve a man and a woman or two partners of the same sex.

Q: What is **sexual health**?

A: There isn't a broadly accepted definition of sexual health because the opinion leaders who have tried to frame this issue often come at it from very different angles. Some focus on the absence of disease or the correct functioning of the reproductive system—the ability to create life and give birth if one chooses to do so. Others place priority on the individual's ability to be comfortable with and take enjoyment from **sexuality**.

An integrated approach to sexual health has all of these elements. We like the definition of sexual health posed by one of the leading nonprofit organizations in the field, the Sex Information and Education Council of the United States (SIECUS). Sexual health, says SIECUS, encompasses not only reproductive health but also the ability to appreciate one's own body, to interact with both genders in respectful ways and to express affection, love and intimacy in ways consistent with one's own values.

SEXUAL HEALTH AND SOCIETY

Q: Aren't we, as a society, overly concerned with sex in some ways?

A: In some ways, perhaps so. The point has often been made in reference to our entertainment industry—the disproportionate amount of sexual content in film and television. We see sex used to sell everything from cosmetics to cars, and sex is often the key to the story line as well. We also are obsessed with youth, and the young adult's exuberant pursuit of sex in its most physical manifestation is disproportionately portrayed. One study showed that a viewer will encounter an average of 22 sexual references in an hour of prime-time TV for every one reference to birth control or disease prevention. Another showed that there were more than eight sexual interactions on average in TV's "family hour."

All of this creates the impression that everyone is having lots of fun with sex and very few problems—especially very few health problems. However, the definitive National Health and Social Life Survey published in 1994 found much evidence to the contrary: Sexual relationships in real life don't much resemble sex on the tube. Americans average fewer than five partners in the course of a lifetime, and they do, of course, have to contend with issues such as **sexually transmitted diseases (STDs)** and unintended or ill-timed pregnancy, as well as problems of sexual function, which can block people from enjoying sex or being able to conceive a child. Far from being overly concerned about these problems, we have failed to give them sufficient attention.

Q: Are significant numbers of people affected by sexual health problems?

A: The numbers are substantial. Take sexually transmitted diseases, for example. If you consider all of the individuals affected by the top 10 reported diseases in the United States, 87 *percent* represent cases of STDs. According to the Institute of Medicine (IOM), the odds of acquiring an STD during a lifetime are one in four, and the rates of many such infections are far higher in this country than any other industrialized nation.

Unintended pregnancy has a similar profile. A million teenage girls become pregnant in the United States every year; about 40 percent of them have **abortions**. According to the Alan Guttmacher Institute, roughly half of all pregnancies in the United States are unintended.

Q: Aren't these essentially issues for the young?

A: Not always. One of the most common STDs, for example, is **genital herpes**. And with herpes, more people are infected between the ages of 25 and 35 than are infected between the ages of 15 and 25. Another example: Forty-two percent of the pregnancies occurring among women between the ages of 30 and 34 are unintended.

This is not to deny the basic point that sexual health is often elusive for the young and that sexual health problems can be tragic. Three million of the estimated 12 million new cases of STDs each year are found among teenagers, and young people are increasingly filling the ranks of those infected with viral diseases such as genital herpes and **genital warts**. Rates of herpes, in particular, have doubled among young adults in the last 10 years alone. And the virus that causes genital warts was found in 60 percent of female students during a three-year Rutgers University study.

Q: Why are the STD rates so high in the United States?

A: An expert panel convened by the IOM published a lengthy report in 1997 that called for a massive national effort to combat what it called the "hidden epidemic" of STDs. The report blamed the STD problem in the United States on a number of factors, including the following:

- Weakness of school-based sex education programs
- Generally low level of public awareness and knowledge
- Lack of training on STDs in medical schools
- Failure to promote STD prevention messages (including **condom** advertising on television)
- Limited access to health care for all segments of the population.

The IOM stressed that sexuality—in spite of our obsession with it—remains something of a taboo topic in many social contexts. People often have trouble finding the words to use when talking to a partner about using condoms, for example, or asking a doctor for information about sex. This reticence contributes to the spread of STDs.

Also, our public health authorities have been unable to exert sufficient political pressure for more direct steps such as condom promotion on television and radio. In most European countries, on the other hand, such messages are broadcast routinely.

Q: Do these same factors contribute to the problem of unintended pregnancy?

A: Education and access to health care services are both critical factors in lowering the rate of teen pregnancies and unintended pregnancies in general. There is good news in that teen pregnancy is on the decline among some segments of the population, yet the United States remains the developed nation with the highest teen pregnancy rate. We provide little sex education, and when we do, it is often in the context of **abstinence**.

In addition, even the informed health consumer faces what might be seen as needless obstacles to acquiring help with family planning. Many insurance companies and managed care organizations, for example, do not cover commonly used birth control methods. According to a survey by the Planned Parenthood Federation of America, 97 percent of health insurance plans cover prescription drugs, but only 33 percent include birth control pills in that coverage. This has forced advocacy organizations to try to compel such coverage through legislation. Meanwhile, the new oral medication for men with problems of sexual function is already covered by some health insurance plans, but research toward a male birth control pill is years away from the market.

Q: But what about so-called sexual function: Do people really need help enjoying sex?

A: Let's look at the facts: When asked about the last 12 months, significant numbers of men and women in one study reported an issue related to sexual performance. Twenty-four percent of women, for example, were unable to reach orgasm with their partners; 17 percent of men had anxiety about their sexual performance; and 15 percent of women suffered pain during sexual activity. The list goes on.

We don't mean to suggest that sexuality in America is a miserable wasteland. In fact, the same survey shows that the majority of people are perfectly happy on the whole with their sexual relationships and have no major medical or psychological problems related to their reproductive and sexual health. All the same, most of us probably encounter some challenges to our sexual health over the course of a lifetime, many of which have to do with various stages of life—pregnancy, parenting, **menopause** and so on. As for sexual function, there are numerous problems that affect sexual performance for tens of millions of Americans every year, including depression and chronic illnesses such as diabetes. The recent launch of a drug to help men have erections caused the biggest sales boom in pharmaceutical history—telling evidence that this is an area where lots of individuals and couples need some help.

Q: **Are sexual health problems in the United States largely a result of the so-called sexual revolution of the 1960s and 1970s?**

A: Some are. Advances in technology such as the birth control pill for women contributed to the trend in which young people felt more free to have sex outside of marriage. This increase in sexual activity, along with a decrease in condom use, clearly led to the steep rise in some sexually transmitted diseases. But many of the issues we list here have been with us for decades. Teen pregnancy, for example, is hardly a recent phenomenon: Our country's highest teen birth rate actually occurred in 1956, a time when many teen pregnancies culminated in the proverbial "shotgun wedding." And as veteran sex educators such as Ruth Westheimer, Ed.D., attest, the problems of sexual function that worry couples today are little different from those at issue 30 years ago: Can a man control his **ejaculation**? Can a woman reach orgasm? Can a man perform sexually as he ages? Is **intercourse** painful? What has changed, according to Westheimer, is that we have a greater degree of openness about sexuality today—perhaps not always in the most constructive way, but openness all the same. This gives us the potential to address some of our most widespread sexual health problems.

Q: **Are people having sex earlier now than they used to?**

A: That is the trend, though it's more gradual than most people realize. For men and women born between 1933 and 1942, the average age at first intercourse was 18. For those born 20 years later, the average age had fallen by about six months. Looked at another way, however, teenage sexual activity *is* on the increase. Between 1971 and 1988, the number of high school seniors who had had more than one sexual partner increased by nearly 60 percent.

Q: Why the change?

A: In reality, there are biological as well as cultural factors at play in this trend. Due to improved health and nutrition, children reach puberty at earlier ages than they used to. At the turn of the century, the average age for onset of puberty for girls was 17; today, it's 11. Meanwhile, the average age at which people marry has also changed. Some 80 percent of those born between 1933 and 1942 had married by age 27 versus 50 percent among those born 20 years later. This makes it more likely for Americans today to have had several sexual partners before they settle into a marriage or another long-term relationship.

Q: Whatever happened to the old rule that you "wait until you're married"?

A: With all that we see and think about a promiscuous society, it is noteworthy that some 16 percent of men and 20 percent of women still remain virgins until marriage. Whether it is best to remain sexually abstinent before entering a lifelong commitment is probably debatable because the decision is more a matter of religious and cultural values than medical fact. There is no debate that abstinence before marriage gives a couple the best chance to avoid sexually transmitted diseases.

Nevertheless, it's important to acknowledge that sexual health is not merely a matter of avoiding disease. Equally important is the ability to appreciate one's body and to express love and intimacy in ways that are mutually satisfying.

Q: Is having sex as a teenager harmful?

A: Not necessarily, but there are obviously some problems with this trend. We've already mentioned STD rates and teen pregnancy, and there are psychological issues as well. The motivation to start having sex is not always straightforward. In some surveys, more than half of adolescent girls report that they did not want to have intercourse the first time but went along with it anyway. And we're now finding that a growing number of boys feel the same way.

The classic double standard places our children in an awkward position. Sexual prowess—even promiscuity—is considered desirable in the young man, but virginity or "purity" is still the desired quality for young women. Yet these same young women must compete for boys' attention as a measure of self-worth, often having to resort to sex out of peer pressure rather than desire. This social context does not help our young people develop a healthy concept of sexuality that hinges on mutual respect and an ability to express intimacy without violating their values. To reach this goal, we need to create a more informed and intelligent dialogue about a range of sexual health issues.

SEX AND HEALTH: REFRAMING THE DIALOGUE

Q: **How can we help bring about a long-term change in our approach to sexuality and sexual health?**

A: Our children represent the key opportunity, but the change starts with us. Adults need to begin to have better insights into their own sexuality—why they do the things they do, what they believe, why they have insecurities—and they need to translate this awareness into a better approach to the next generation.

At an institutional level, we have to make our health care system more sensitive to sexual health needs—and make this a routine part of care. And we have to give people the education to make them more aggressive in taking care of these issues. Some of that starts in the home, and some starts in the school.

Q: **What about the role of the medical establishment? If so many people are affected, aren't these problems dealt with routinely in the doctor's office?**

A: Not by a long shot. Many researchers note serious obstacles to providing quality care for issues of sexual health. A 1992 survey of primary care physicians by the Centers for Disease Control and Prevention (CDC), for example, found that the taking of a basic sexual history was anything but routine. Only 49 percent of physicians surveyed asked new adult patients about STDs, 31 percent asked about condom use and 22 percent about the number of sex partners. By contrast, 94 percent of physicians asked patients about cigarette smoking. Perhaps cigarette smoking is an easier topic to broach than pain during intercourse or failure to reach orgasm, but all of these issues are important.

In fairness to health care professionals, many people are embarrassed to mention sexual health problems, so there is some reluctance on the part of the doctor *and* the patient to open a dialogue about sexual health. In addition, most M.D.'s have received miserably few hours of education about sexually transmitted diseases and even less about issues of sexual function. Without this training, health care professionals bring just as many prejudices and value judgments to a patient consultation as anyone else.

Q: **How can the health care system do a better job on sexual health issues?**

A: The first thing is to ask that very question. Unfortunately, up until now, sexual health per se really hasn't been on the list of priorities for either the private or public sector. Until we acknowledge that it has more importance, we won't do more about it. Second, we need to begin to see sexual health as a more integral part of our physical and mental wellness. More than simply the absence of disease, it should be a source of joy and fulfillment. Third, we need to make men accountable for their share of the work in improving the collective reproductive and sexual health.

Q: **Why men?**

A: That may seem like an odd statement, but consider the facts: Family planning in this country is organized around women (as in "women's clinics"), the most popular methods of birth control are female-controlled, and women, obviously, bear the children. For all of these reasons, women must seek regular medical care focused specifically on reproductive, if not sexual, health. Why don't we have contraceptive methods for men?

Sexually transmitted infections offer another case in point. Because of their anatomy, women are more likely to acquire STDs and suffer the worst consequences of these sorts of infections. For example, as we explain in chapter 3, one of the most common STDs is a virus that plays a role in cancer of the **cervix**. Women are advised to get regular tests—in the form of **Pap smears**—

for this virus. Men, clearly, play a role in spreading the virus, but suggestions that men be routinely tested have fallen on deaf ears. Nor, strictly speaking, do men have the equivalent of a gynecologist or women's health specialist. So the burden continues to fall on women.

FIRST IMPRESSIONS OF SEXUAL HEALTH

Q: You talk about the problems of youth and the pressures young people face. When should parents start talking with children about sex?

A: A healthy concept of sexuality begins early. Parents should *start* talking about sex, according to many behavioral experts, whenever children ask or the issue comes up. With the approach often recommended today, information about sex is not delivered in the kind of formal parent-child session that we used to think of as "the talk" but rather in a long series of fairly routine conversations. When parents avoid the subject, children get the idea that sexuality is indeed something they should be embarrassed about—or else something they don't want to talk to Mom or Dad about. The open approach, by contrast, is supposed to create a feeling that sexual development is a normal part of growing up—and that parents can be a good source of information and guidance on everything from early feelings of attraction and love to reproductive health decisions.

Q: Is there evidence that talking about sex in the home will make kids more likely to have sex at earlier ages and put themselves at risk?

A: Much of the evidence is to the contrary. Young people who discuss sexuality issues with parents have been shown to be more likely to postpone intercourse and more likely to use contraceptives when they do become sexually active.

In reality, parents are their children's first sex ed teachers, whether or not they ever mention the word. The impressions parents convey about body image, physical affection, gender roles and privacy are the beginnings of sexual awareness.

Parents' opportunities, however, are not limitless. As a survey by the Kaiser Family Foundation showed in 1997, most 10- to 12-year-olds rated parents an important source on issues, including sex and AIDS. Teens, however, were more likely to name friends than parents. This emphasizes the importance of starting early.

Q: What's the role of school-based sex education? Does it help? Or is there a case to be made that school-based sex education is driving down the age of first sexual activity?

A: This is an issue about which there is great debate. The political demise of former U.S. Surgeon General Joycelyn Elders, M.D., is just one testimony to the controversy surrounding that issue.

We believe that school-based programs can have a positive role. And whatever else one can say, it seems overwhelmingly clear at this point that the trend to increased sexual activity in adolescence has taken place *in spite of* relatively little sex education in the classroom. For example, it's estimated that by the time he finishes 12th grade, the average American child has been exposed to about 11,000 hours of school curricula. Of this time, only a fraction is devoted to health education generally, and sexuality is often dispensed with in less than a week. In fact, less than 10 percent of American school children get comprehensive sex education.

By comparison, the average high school graduate has watched 15,000 to 20,000 hours of television. Many studies have shown that the sexual content of television represents a large part of what passes for sex education, and some research indicates that TV is the leading source of sexuality information for teens.

Q: How do the media affect young people's attitudes about sexuality?

A: We've already mentioned the heavy emphasis on sexual content on television, and behavioral scientists have also documented the impact on adolescent sexual development of media such as popular music, movies and magazines. The consensus among many researchers is that all of these media too often purvey messages that glorify sex and, in particular, sexualize girls, inducing them to judge themselves by how they look rather than by how they think, feel or solve problems. In a survey conducted by researchers at Radcliffe, adolescent girls complained that there was too much sex on television. Even preadolescent girls felt pressure to make themselves look sexy.

Q: In what way do girls feel more pressure than boys?

A: The national fixation with body image, fueled by the average teenager's exposure to some 20,000 television advertisements per year, creates special pressures for girls in several ways. A study that analyzed TV, movies and magazines found a dramatic emphasis on physical appearance, with women being two to three times more likely to make or receive comments about their appearance than men. And the standard of attractiveness for women centers on a body type that is at best uncommon. More than half of boys and nearly two-thirds of girls say the female characters they see on TV are thinner than women in real life, whereas men are portrayed more realistically. Perhaps this shouldn't be surprising when the average model is five foot nine and weighs 110 pounds—five inches taller and 32 pounds lighter than the average American woman. The outcome for girls can involve not only emotional distress but also health problems: Some 31 percent of nine-year-olds think they're too fat, and 11 percent of high school students have eating disorders.

Q: Is the role of the media all bad?

A: Not really. The same powerful influence can and sometimes is applied in a more positive direction. An increasing number of programs—both general-audience and youth-oriented shows—portray women as capable and effective for their work and talent, as well as for their looks. And several organizations concerned with sexual health are now working with producers, scriptwriters, directors and others to develop more realistic and more positive portrayals of sexual relationships.

The mass media certainly are capable of opening our eyes to pressing sexuality issues, as evidenced by the successful AIDS awareness campaigns of the 1980s and by the major impact of television shows such as "Ellen," which took on the formerly taboo subject of sexual orientation.

UNDERSTANDING GENDER AND SEXUAL ORIENTATION

Q: What is meant by the term "sexual orientation"?

A: Sexual orientation, or sexual identity, refers to the way that women and men identify their most profound sexual attractions. In broad terms, an attraction to a person of the same sex is termed **homosexuality**; an attraction to a person of the opposite sex is **heterosexuality**. While these are the predominant categories in our society, it's widely acknowledged that some individuals find themselves drawn sexually to both sexes, an orientation referred to as **bisexuality**.

In his pioneering studies, sexuality researcher Alfred Kinsey, Sc.D., introduced as a theoretical model a continuum of sexual orientation (see box) that allowed for the fact that some of us are attracted solely to the opposite sex, some solely to the same sex and some, in varying degrees, to both sexes. The Kinsey continuum helped to pave the way for a less monolithic view of sexual orientation, in which both homosexuality and bisexuality are seen as a part of the breadth of human sexuality.

The Kinsey Scale

0 = Exclusively heterosexual

1 = Predominantly heterosexual, only incidentally homosexual

2 = Predominantly heterosexual, but more than incidentally homosexual

3 = Equally heterosexual and homosexual

4 = Predominantly homosexual, but more than incidentally heterosexual

5 = Predominantly homosexual, but incidentally heterosexual

6 = Exclusively homosexual

Reprinted by permission of The Kinsey Institute for Research in Sex, Gender and Reproduction, Inc., from *Sexual Behavior in the Human Male* (1948) by Alfred C. Kinsey.

Recently, it has been suggested that these tendencies may change over time, with people expressing bisexual tendencies at one point in their lives and heterosexuality or homosexuality at another.

Q: Is sexual orientation determined biologically, or is it a matter of social conditioning?

A: Research suggests that sexual orientation is a largely biological function. There is, for example, a study of twins separated at birth who both turned out to be homosexual despite having been raised in totally different environments. Further, geneticists have located a gene that is allegedly linked to male homosexuality, and some neuroscientists believe that there are differences in the brain that may account for a physiological basis to sexual orientation.

This field of research is far from complete, and there may prove to be cultural influences as well. Yet in behavioral studies, many homosexual men and women report that they have a clear sense of same-sex attraction at an early age. In addition, children raised by same-sex parents are no more likely to have a homosexual orientation than children raised by a man and woman.

Q: Does that mean bisexuality is a biological condition?

A: Attitudes toward bisexuality are an interesting case in point. Some prefer to think that a person must be either homosexual or heterosexual, and that anyone who claims to be bisexual is making a choice to indulge in something that has no physiological basis. But as the Kinsey Scale suggests, some people find themselves strongly attracted to both sexes and report feeling frustrated by social norms that characterize this as a self-indulgent or deliberately rebellious choice.

Q: How many people are gay or bisexual?

A: Experts on sexual behavior believe no study has ever provided a totally credible answer. In the National Health and Social Life Survey, which was mentioned earlier, less than 5 percent of men and women identified themselves as bisexual or homosexual. Slightly larger percentages reported having same-sex fantasies. Many of those who work in this area of research, however, point out that the strong stigma associated with homosexuality skews the accuracy of such surveys.

Q: Can you tell me what is meant by the terms "**transsexual**" and "**cross-dresser**"?

A: The transsexual is someone who views his gender as being the opposite of what anatomy would normally dictate: someone born with male genitals, for example, who feels he is instead a woman. Transsexuals often use medications or surgeries to alter their bodies, and they may also choose to wear clothing of the gender they have identified as being consistent with their essential nature. Far more common is cross-dressing, or **transvestism**, which simply means dressing in the clothes of the opposite sex. Cross-dressing is a behavior associated with both men and women and with all sexual orientations. It can be a form of caricature, a sort of ritual or an attempt to attract members of the same sex.

PATTERNS OF SEXUAL BEHAVIOR

Q: What is considered the peak age for sexual drive?

A: Even though both sexes become biologically prepared for sexual activity during adolescence, men tend to be most orgasmic during adolescence and in their early 20s. Women tend to be most orgasmic between their mid-20s and mid-40s. The reasons for this are complex: As compared with boys, adolescent girls are less likely to experiment with sexual response by masturbating. Women tend to feel more comfortable with their sexuality as they mature, and by their 40s, they are often buoyed by enhanced self-confidence and a much reduced fear of pregnancy, to name just a couple of factors.

Q: What is the peak age for fertility?

A: Women experience **ovulation** (the monthly release of eggs) most regularly between the ages of 18 and 28, which means it's easier for them to get pregnant during these years. Men can manufacture **sperm** anytime after puberty, but the number of sperm produced is thought to be highest between the ages of 21 and 30.

Studies show that 40 percent of problems with **fertility**—the ability to conceive a child—are related to the male partner, 40 percent are related to the female partner and 20 percent are of unknown origin or are related to both partners.

Q: How often do most people have sexual intercourse?

A: Rates vary tremendously. The National Health and Social Life Survey found that about 35 percent of respondents had sex more than two times per week, about 35 percent had sex one or several times a month, and the remaining 30 percent had sex a few times a year or not at all.

Overall, about a third of married couples have sex two or three times a week. Interestingly, this is higher than the rate among singles who don't live with a partner and lower than the rate among singles with a live-in mate. Couples who identify themselves as gay or bisexual, according to the researchers, engage in sexual activity at roughly the same rates, though gay and bisexual singles have relatively higher numbers of partners.

Q: Is the frequency of sex with a partner an important indicator of sexual health?

A: Frequency is an issue for many couples. One of the most common reasons that couples see a sex therapist is a mismatch of sexual desire—one partner's feeling that the other has lost interest in sex. On the other hand, frequency is not nearly as meaningful an index of satisfaction as one might think. Sexual drive and expression are probably as unique as the proverbial fingerprint, and a person having sex once a week may be as happy and healthy as someone who engages in sex five times as often. The important thing is to make sure both partners agree on the frequency of intercourse and talk about what to do if they don't.

Q: Does sexual activity decline markedly as people age?

A: Contrary to popular belief, people can continue to have satisfying sexual relationships for as long as they want. In studies of sexual activity among those over 60, researchers find, not surprisingly, that those who enjoy sex in their 30s and 40s tend to continue to share satisfying sex into their 70s and 80s. Those who find sex distasteful in their younger years or have sexual health problems often see old age as a way of closing this chapter of their lives or relationships.

Sexual drive, on the other hand, does lessen with age, and both men and women can experience a loss of sexual function, including problems associated with changing levels of **hormones**. Medical science, however, has devised a growing array of treatments for problems of sexual function. We talk about these in chapter 2.

For the most part, those over age 60, whether single or in couples, continue to have an interest in sex and often become more comfortable and more open with one another.

Q: Is oral sex normal?

A: Yes. At some time in their lives, about three-quarters of women and men have both given and received oral sex. Not everyone enjoys it, however. While 45 percent of men find receiving oral sex "very appealing," only 17 percent of women say the same about giving it. And 29 percent of women say that receiving oral sex is "very appealing"—while 34 percent of men say the same about giving it.

Q: What percentage of people have anal intercourse?

A: Roughly one-quarter of men and one-fifth of women say they have experimented with anal sex at some point. Far fewer—less than 10 percent—report having had anal intercourse in the last year.

Q: How many people masturbate?

A: More than 60 percent of men and nearly half of all women masturbate. Women tend to start masturbating at a later age than men, and they masturbate less often: 27 percent of men masturbate once a week, compared with only 8 percent of women.

It's important to note that masturbation is not a singles-only phenomenon: A large percentage of those who live with a partner—85 percent of men and 45 percent of women—say they masturbate. Married people, in fact, are significantly more likely to masturbate than those living alone. About half of those surveyed felt guilty about masturbation.

Q: Does masturbation desensitize the sexual organs or have other ill effects?

A: This is a question that many people pose, apparently out of worries that self-pleasuring is either psychologically unhealthy or a potential medical problem. The fact is that most of us grow up with the idea that masturbation is at least embarrassing or possibly morally wrong in some way. Some religious traditions, for example, frown on it. Yet, as is evident from the number of people who do masturbate, the practice is a normal part of sexual discovery and exploration.

Masturbation can be beneficial physiologically: As one ages, for example, it can help keep pelvic muscles toned. It can also be extremely useful in helping men and women learn more about their patterns of arousal so that they can relax and enjoy sex with a partner. This aspect of self-pleasuring is discussed in chapter 2.

Occasionally, masturbation can become compulsive and have detrimental effects on a relationship. Frequent masturbation may interfere with a person's ability to be aroused by a partner, leaving both with unsatisfactory sexual experiences. In addition, a small number of people may develop habitual ways of masturbating and become dependent on these for orgasm. This may lead to problems adapting their "style" to sex with a partner.

Q: How many people use **vibrators**? Are they harmful?

A: In the largest survey to date, an estimated 2 percent of sexually active American adults use vibrators either for partnered sex or masturbation, and 1 percent say they use other sex toys.

While many types of vibrators are not made for insertion into the **vagina** or **anus**, some are, and these devices can cause internal damage if they are used improperly. We talk about vibrators and safety in chapter 2.

ACHIEVING SEXUAL HEALTH

Q: Speaking of safety, what is meant by the term "**safer sex**"?

A: The term became popular in the 1980s largely because of the major public awareness campaigns about the AIDS epidemic and the need to protect oneself or one's partner from sexually transmitted diseases. Safer sex refers to any measure taken to limit the spread of infection from one person to another. This can include changes in intimate behavior and use of barriers such as condoms that block the exchange of body fluids, both of which are discussed in chapter 3.

Taking responsibility for STD prevention is a vital concept for people of all sexual orientations, all ages, all races—a fundamental part of sexual health.

For heterosexuals, however, there is another critical issue that goes hand in hand with disease prevention—the prevention of unwanted pregnancy. A thorough approach to safer sex would begin with **contraception**, the measures one takes to prevent unplanned pregnancy. We discuss this in detail in chapter 5.

Q: Do contraceptives help to prevent sexually transmitted diseases?

A: Barriers such as condoms, **diaphragms** and **spermicides** do offer varying degrees of protection against infectious diseases spread during sex. Unfortunately, many people presume that any form of birth control will make sex "safe," and this is not at all true. Someone who is using the birth control pill—indeed, most forms of birth control—is still at risk of infectious diseases. That's why people need to make careful choices, taking precautions that address the potential needs for both birth control and STD prevention.

Q: Will safer sex result in sexual health?

A: Only in the most limited sense. The concept of prevention is vital, but sexual health is more than the absence of disease. In its fullest sense, it requires an acceptance of sexuality as a potential source of joy and fulfillment. Many of our cultural assumptions reflect a negative attitude towards sexuality—a preoccupation with loss of purity, risk of pregnancy, risk of disease, a fall from grace. Unfortunately, as a consequence, we fail to keep in perspective the notion that sexuality is a basic part of our makeup—and vital to our physical and emotional health.

Q: Is there really any evidence that sexual health has a direct bearing on overall health and happiness?

A: Actually, there is. In the comprehensive National Health and Social Life Survey, researchers found several remarkable correlations between the status of sexual relationships and perceptions of physical health and happiness. For example, those with a steady partner were more likely to rate themselves as "extremely happy" or "very happy" than those without one, and the same was true of those who had sex several times a week versus those who didn't. In addition, those reporting a problem with sexual function such as difficulty reaching orgasm or having pain during sex were less likely than others to describe their health status as "excellent" or "good" than others.

Findings such as these, of course, don't fully establish cause and effect, but they suggest that sexual expression is integrally linked with our general sense of fulfillment and well-being. And this holds true to clinical experience, in which sexual health problems are not mere details that can be swept under the carpet. Instead, they are issues that demand attention because of their impact on intimate relationships and on self-esteem.

Q: So how do I become sexually healthy?

A: The first point is to realize not only that you *can* take pleasure and fulfillment from your sexuality but that you also *deserve* to take it. Too often, physicians see women resign themselves to a life without sexual pleasure, wrongly assuming that their inability to achieve orgasm was all in their heads. They also see men live with impotence (and their marriages dissolve) because they were too embarrassed to ask for help. Because of these experiences, it's clear to us that sexuality is an area where we need to apply the popular term "empowerment." Too many people with legitimate sexual health problems do not get help either because of the stigma that surrounds frank discussion of sex in real life or because the health care system fails to recognize the importance of the person's complaint. One step to this empowerment is information, and by educating yourself through books such as this one, you are taking a vital step.

2 SEXUAL FUNCTION: TAKING PLEASURE FROM SEX

THE MECHANICS OF AROUSAL

Q: What triggers sexual arousal?

A: The process of sexual arousal is a body-mind response triggered by any signal that we interpret as erotic. To attempt to catalog all of the things that a person might find arousing is a futile task given the enormous range of our sexual desires and appetites. To generalize, many of these signals are functions of the senses—a touch, for example, or a particular smell or visual cue. Others have to do entirely with internal stimuli—a fantasy or memory, for instance.

Whatever the trigger, researchers believe that the process of arousal centers on chemical "messengers" known as **neurotransmitters**, which are involved in virtually every human function. These chemicals—moving back and forth along nerve pathways between the brain, spinal cord and genitals—set into motion the physical changes that we experience as sexual readiness.

Q: What sorts of physical changes are typical?

A: In broad strokes, there are two major engines of physiological response. The first is **vasocongestion**, an increased flow of blood in various parts of the body, particularly the **penis** and outer portion of the vagina. The second is a process in which neurotransmitters produce heightened levels of neuromuscular tension—more energy in the nerves and muscles.

As a result of these two responses, we may experience heightened sensitivity anywhere from the fingertips to the lips to the genital organs. The most widely used framework for understanding the workings of the body during a sexual encounter, known as the **sexual response cycle**, comes from the famous sex researchers William H. Masters, M.D., a gynecologist, and Virginia E. Johnson, a psychologist. They describe the physiological process by dividing it into four stages: **excitement**, **plateau**, orgasm and **resolution**.

Q: How does a man's body respond during the excitement phase?

A: Heart rate and muscle tension increase. Nipples may become erect, and other parts of the body may become highly sensitive to touch. One of the early signs of arousal in many men is **erection**, the process through which the penis becomes rigid enough for penetrative intercourse.

Q: How exactly does the penis become erect?

A: The penis consists of soft tissue—not muscle, as some have been given to believe—that is crisscrossed with nerves and blood vessels. Through the center of the penis runs the **urethra**, the canal through which urine is carried out of the body from the **bladder**. Around it are arrayed three spongy, tubelike structures that largely comprise the shaft of the penis. Two are called the corpora cavernosa; the other is the corpus spongiosum. As blood flow increases during the excitement phase, the spongy tissue becomes engorged and expands, causing the penis to become firm and, to varying degrees, erect. The firmness of erection varies greatly during lovemaking depending on the kind of stimulation being exchanged between partners.

Q: What's the role of the testes in sexual function? Are they part of the arousal process?

A: The testes, or testicles, are organs that play two critical functions in sex and reproduction: First, they set the stage for all sexual activity by manufacturing the hormone **testosterone**, which at puberty triggers the development of the mature male body. After puberty, testosterone helps to maintain sexual drive.

Second, the testes manufacture sperm, the male's contribution to the reproductive act. A sperm cell is microscopic, approximately 0.05 millimeter long and shaped like a tadpole, with a long tail that literally helps it to swim in the environment of the vagina where it attempts to reach and fertilize an egg. Sperm are produced in the testes at a rate of about 100 million a day and take about 70 days to mature. Sperm mature in tightly coiled tubing inside the testes called the **epididymis** and travel to the urethra through a canal called the **vas deferens**. (An illustration of the male reproductive system can be found in the appendix of this book.)

During the excitement stage of sexual response, the testes are drawn in more tightly to the body, and the **scrotum**, the sack of skin that holds the testes, becomes thicker and firmer.

Q: So what's next—what is plateau like for men?

A: "Plateau" is perhaps an odd choice of words for the second stage of sexual response, given that many of our sexual reflexes simply increase at this point. If stimulation continues—from kissing, caressing, penetration or any other form of sex play—erection usually becomes more rigid; the testes become enlarged and are pulled in even closer; heart rate and blood pressure continue to rise; and muscular tension waxes. Researchers also have noted that many people—ironically, in the midst of this sensory feast—suffer diminished hearing and vision. Finally, about one-quarter of men experience what's known as **sex flush**, pink or red blotches typically found around the breasts or elsewhere on the upper body.

Q: How long does plateau last? What pushes a man to orgasm?

A: Patterns of sexual arousal are highly variable, and a sexual encounter might last anywhere from minutes to an hour or more. The process is seldom a straight trajectory of escalating arousal. Distractions, awkward positions, an uncomfortable touch—any of these can cause a momentary waning of pleasure or loss of erection. Sometimes sexual partners do not reach orgasm at all, as we discuss later in this chapter. Often, however, they recover quickly from these disruptions and continue stimulation until neuromuscular tension builds to the point where one or both reach the edge of orgasm.

In men, this moment is marked by a sort of "point of no return" called **ejaculatory inevitability**, meaning that the man is now certain to have an orgasm and to ejaculate.

Q: What exactly is meant by the term "ejaculate"?

A: To ejaculate—as it applies to men—is to expel sperm and other fluids from the male reproductive organs through the urethral opening at the tip of the penis. Understanding the sequence of events that leads to ejaculation requires knowing a bit more about the male reproductive system—the plumbing, as it were.

Sperm don't make the journey from the testes through the penis all by themselves. Instead, they are carried in a fluid called **semen**, which in turn requires secretions from three internal organs: the **prostate gland**, the two **Cowper's glands** and the **seminal vesicles** (see appendix of this book).

During plateau, the Cowper's glands secrete a clear fluid, which enters and lubricates the urethra. The prostate is a small, doughnut-shaped gland that surrounds the urethra where it joins the bladder. The prostate, too, secretes a fluid, and at the threshold of orgasm, a series of contractions move this fluid to join with secretions of the third key organ, the seminal vesicles.

The seminal vesicles are, in effect, a basin. In this basin are joined the sperm that have traveled through the vas deferens and the secretions from the prostate and seminal vesicles themselves. All of these mix and then pass into the urethra as semen.

Q: So ejaculatory inevitability leads to orgasm?

A: Yes. What a man feels at the point of ejaculatory inevitability is a pooling of semen at the urethral opening that is brought on by contractions in the prostate, the seminal vesicles and vas deferens at the threshold of orgasm. Next comes orgasm: a second series of contractions less than a second apart in the urethra and penis. The contractions expel semen through the urethral opening, where it gushes or drips out, depending on the strength of the contractions.

Q: Can a man have an orgasm and not ejaculate?

A: Some men can experience orgasmic contractions and whole-body pleasure without ejaculating, but it's not common. Special exercises may be needed in order for a man to attain this extraordinary level of muscle control.

Q: OK, so what about women? What happens in a woman's body during the excitement phase of sexual arousal?

A: The same processes of vasocongestion and neuromuscular tension are at work, bringing about changes that in some ways closely parallel those in men, such as sex flush (which is more common in women than in men) and erect nipples. Heart rate quickens, muscles respond, and blood begins to rush to various parts of the body, including the breasts, the **vulva** and the vagina.

Q: What exactly is the difference between the vagina and vulva?

A: The vulva refers to the external genitals, including the **clitoris**, urethra, the vaginal lips (**labia majora** [outer lips] and **labia minora** [inner lips]) and the vaginal opening itself. The vagina, strictly speaking, is an internal organ, a small tube about three to four inches long surrounded by muscle and lined with mucous membranes such as those found in the mouth or anus. The vagina is bordered at its rear by the cervix, the opening to the **uterus**, which is the expandable internal organ where a fetus will grow and develop before birth. The opening of the vagina is sometimes called the introitus. (Illustrations of the female reproductive system can be found in the appendix of this book.)

Q: So how are the vagina and vulva affected by sexual excitement?

A: One of the first changes is wetness in the vagina, also termed **lubrication**. This parallels erection in some ways—it's the direct result of vasocongestion in the walls of the vagina, causing fluid that is stored in the vaginal lining to seep through. Lubrication is also provided by the **Bartholin's glands**, small glands located in the vulva near the opening of the vagina. Lubrication is a gradual process and may not be noticeable until the fluid begins to gather and trickle towards the vaginal opening.

Meanwhile, the expandable interior of the vagina becomes deeper and wider.

In the vulva, the labia minora will thicken, and the labia majora will open back to expose more of the vaginal opening. In addition, the clitoris will become firmer and more sensitive, and it will pull back until it is under its hood.

Q: Can you tell me more about the clitoris? Some people say it's the key to sexual arousal in women.

A: Patterns of sexual response are highly individual, as we discuss throughout this chapter. But the clitoris is without doubt the premier center of stimulation in most women. It's a small, round gland at the very top of the vulva with the sole function of providing sexual pleasure. The clitoral hood, which we mentioned earlier, is connected to the vaginal lips. In vaginal intercourse, the penis moves in and out of the vagina and tugs on the labia, causing indirect clitoral stimulation. The size of the clitoris and its distance from the vagina vary from woman to woman. Depending on the size and position of the clitoris and its hood, direct stimulation may be needed. However, direct stimulation should be approached carefully since the clitoris can become hypersensitive when aroused.

Q: How does a woman respond in the plateau phase?

A: A key sign of plateau in women is a marked swelling of the walls in the outer third of the vagina (near the vaginal opening), a phenomenon called the **orgasmic platform**. As Masters and Johnson note, in vaginal intercourse, this nerve-rich platform can effectively grasp the shaft of a penis, whatever its size.

Lubrication continues during the plateau phase but may wax and wane as does an erection. The inner two-thirds of the vagina expand further in width and depth. And the clitoris enlarges but pulls back against the pubic bone. This, together with the swelling of the vaginal lips, makes it harder to locate beneath the clitoral hood.

Because of the continued pooling of blood, vaginal lips may turn red, sex flush may intensify and spread, and the area around the nipples may become swollen.

Q: Does a woman experience something equivalent to "ejaculatory inevitability"?

A: No. Although there are many parallels between male and female sexual response, women do not seem to have an equivalent mechanism: A woman can be on the verge of orgasm and be deterred at the last second by any number of distractions or a failure of stimulation.

Q: What is the first sensation of orgasm in a woman?

A: Most women report that their first sensations of orgasm are feelings of intense warmth and pleasure centering on the clitoris, and for most, it is stimulation of the clitoris that brings them to this moment. As in men, orgasm involves a series of involuntary contractions, which in women involve the orgasmic platform, the uterus and the anus.

Q: How else are orgasms different in men and women?

A: Surprisingly, the rate of orgasmic contractions is precisely the same in men as in women—less than a second apart—and sensations at the moment of climax don't differ much either. Written descriptions of orgasm by men and women are virtually identical when no reference is made to anatomy or ejaculation.

One potential difference is ejaculation. As we mentioned earlier, men usually ejaculate when they climax. Most women don't, although some women report having an ejaculation, which may be in some cases a buildup of vaginal secretions that lubricate the vagina during sex and in others a release of urine.

Q: What about **multiple orgasm**?

A: Multiple orgasm is another potential difference. Although fewer than half of orgasmic women have ever had multiple climaxes (generally defined as two or more climaxes per single sex act), many sexologists believe that all women have the *potential* to experience such orgasms. Men, by contrast, are generally said to be less capable of multiple orgasm, though it's not impossible for men.

Q: Why the difference in multiple orgasms?

A: This goes back to the Masters and Johnson model and the final stage of sexual arousal, called resolution. This last phase immediately follows orgasm and consists of the time it takes for the body to return to its unaroused state.

Though both sexes experience resolution after climax, there are certain differences between male and female response. For most men, the resolution phase is also a **refractory period**, lasting at least a few minutes, during which they are unable to have another climax even if the penis is still erect and stimulation continues. Women, though, do not have a refractory period, which means that they have the potential to reenter the plateau stage right after orgasm and have another climax (or several) before reaching resolution.

Some experts say that a small percentage of men apparently lack a refractory period and thus have the ability to be multi-orgasmic. Others can learn to have multiple orgasms, these researchers say, by developing the ability to separate orgasm from ejaculation and thereby have one or more climaxes before ejaculating semen.

Q: Does everyone have orgasms?

A: A small percentage of men—roughly 10 percent—have difficulty reaching orgasm, and anywhere from 25 to 50 percent of women do not climax consistently with intercourse.

PROBLEMS AND CONCERNS FOR WOMEN

Anorgasmia

Q: What would cause a woman to have difficulty reaching orgasm?

A: The inability to reach orgasm—called **anorgasmia**—is a complicated issue that has been studied more in women than men. Most often, its cause relates to anatomy and technique. Most women (according to some research, as many as 75 percent) need direct stimulation of the clitoris to reach climax, and vaginal intercourse simply isn't the best way to provide that.

Other factors can interfere with orgasm, too, such as pain during sex or psychological issues. Research shows this problem sometimes actually relates to a failure to recognize orgasm when it occurs. In other words, some women will physiologically show signs of orgasm when monitored but still report not having orgasm. This may be due in part to unfulfilled expectations—the idea that orgasm must be an overwhelming and dramatic experience even though it is sometimes quite subtle.

Q: How is the clitoris best stimulated?

A: Direct stimulation of the clitoris may take a variety of forms. Most commonly these include oral stimulation of the clitoris with the tongue or lips, called **cunnilingus**, and stimulation with the fingers in place of—or in addition to—penetrative vaginal intercourse.

In addition, couples often need to try a variety of positions for vaginal intercourse in order to determine which will provide the most clitoral stimulation. For example, the so-called missionary position (prone position with the man on top) may be less effective than a woman-on-top position.

Q: Can other kinds of stimulation bring a woman to orgasm?

A: Yes. There is no one-size-fits-all formula for sexual pleasure. Women report having climaxes through many other forms of lovemaking, including caressing or kissing of the breasts. Some report that even fantasy can bring them to climax.

Perhaps the most talked about alternative to clitoral stimulation is stimulation of the **Grafenberg spot (G-spot)**, a cushion of tissue that can be felt an inch or two up on the wall of the vagina toward the stomach. The G-spot is named after German gynecologist Ernst Grafenberg, who was the first to hypothesize that it played a key role in female sexual response. (If a woman is trying to locate the G-spot herself, she may need to squat or lie down and bring her knees up to change the position of her pelvis for easier access.) Researchers disagree on the strength of the scientific evidence for the G-spot, but significant numbers of women report that continuous stimulation of the area can lead to orgasm.

Q: Does it get easier for women to have orgasms when they get older?

A: Yes. According to the 1990 *Kinsey Institute New Report on Sex,* women tend to be most orgasmic in their 40s, while males experience their greatest frequency of orgasm during their teens to early 20s.

Some therapists believe women become more orgasmic later in life because they come to feel more secure about their sexuality and relationships and therefore are better able to explore their sexual responses. While men generally start experimenting with masturbation as adolescents, women are statistically less likely to do so, and studies of adolescence show that girls may focus more on pleasing a partner than maximizing their own pleasure.

Q: What's the recommended therapy for a woman who rarely reaches orgasm?

A: Therapists who work with women on this subject look at a number of different issues, including potential psychological and emotional blocks. Some women—and men—suffer from **anticipatory anxiety:** They want an orgasm so much that they fail to relax, breathe normally and let it happen. Talking through the issue with a partner and a specially trained professional, such as a sex therapist, will probably help. But it's important to stress that anorgasmia is usually not "all in the head," as the conventional wisdom would often dictate. It often has to do instead with an individual woman's physiological response to stimulation or the sexual technique of the couple.

Q: **How do you treat a problem that has to do with physiological response?**

A: In many cases of anorgasmia, it's critical to learn more about your particular process of arousal by breaking out of existing sexual patterns. If you are unable to have an orgasm through vaginal intercourse, for example, try something else. Many therapists recommend that women experiment with masturbation. In fact, research shows that women who masturbate on a regular basis experience more orgasms with their partners than women who don't. The idea is that when masturbating, a woman can take her time in an unpressured situation to discover exactly what forms of stimulation arouse her. Therapists may suggest exercises that include yogalike positions that help relax the body or heighten sensation in certain areas and may also suggest reading erotic literature or engaging in various forms of fantasy to augment the process of arousal. These may include use of sex toys such as vibrators, which provide intense clitoral stimulation and can bring a large percentage of women to climax.

In the context of partnered sex, this experimentation may include the same types of exercises with the aim of discovering which areas are the most sexually arousing. Vibrators can be used as part of these exercises as well. For intercourse, sex therapists stress that experimentation with various positions can show couples how to maximize stimulation. The woman-on-top position, for example, can help women control the angle of penetration to stimulate the clitoris or the G-spot.

Q: **Speaking of experimentation, are vibrators safe?**

A: Used properly, they are quite safe. Electric vibrators have been around since the late nineteenth century and continue to evolve in sophistication and diversity. Vibrators can be found in a variety of retail outlets—everywhere from drug stores to sex boutiques—as well as in specialty catalogs.

Women who have decided to try a vibrator for the first time

might find their options rather overwhelming. And once a woman has made her choice, there is still much to learn about using the device. A book or one of the educational videos on vibrators may be helpful.

Many people assume that vibrators are designed for insertion, but only a portion of the devices work this way. Vibrators that can be inserted, however, do raise safety issues. These vibrators must be cleaned after use to avoid bacterial contamination. Equally important, vibrators that are inserted can become lodged in the vagina or anus if misused.

Q: **I've heard there's a serious downside—that vibrators desensitize you to normal touch. Is this true?**

A: This can be a problem. Vibrators deliver a form of stimulation that can produce orgasms very quickly in some women. For this reason, regular vibrator users sometimes have trouble readjusting to the slower pace of body-to-body pleasuring. In making this transition back to partnered sex, therapists say it's helpful for a woman to adjust her expectations and allow for the fact that arousal will take more time. Gradually, she can become reacquainted with stimulation without a vibrator. Another approach, of course, is to include the vibrator in lovemaking with a partner.

Q: **How can a woman experience the "multiple orgasm" phenomenon?**

A: Clarifying expectations may be the first step. In that spirit, some therapists prefer using the term "serial orgasm" rather than "multiple orgasm" because some women have the expectation that orgasms will follow immediately on top of one another. What's more realistic is to think that a woman can have more than one orgasm in a session with herself or her partner.

The first step is continuing stimulation after the first orgasm, something not every partner will provide. Even if they do have partners who are willing, however, some women don't respond to additional stimulation after an orgasm because the clitoris becomes hypersensitive. The solution may be to wait a few seconds after climaxing, keep breathing rhythmically and then continue with gentler stimulation.

A word of caution: Some experts point out that focusing too much on multiple orgasms tends to be counterproductive and can interfere with sexual pleasure. In the final analysis, a woman's level of sexual satisfaction isn't linked to the number of climaxes she experiences per sex act.

Pain During Intercourse

Q: Is it unusual for a woman to experience physical pain during intercourse?

A: No. **Dyspareunia**, or painful intercourse, is among the most common sexual complaints that women report to their gynecologists. Surveys show that more that 15 percent of women experience physical pain with sex some of the time. Although the causes of dyspareunia are sometimes presumed to be psychological, most often they have to do with physiological problems such as infections, lack of lubrication, issues of technique and anatomic features.

Q: What kinds of infections result in pain during sex?

A: A major proportion of dyspareunia is caused by widespread infections such as **vulvovaginal candidiasis** (more commonly known as a **yeast infection** or **VVC**), which can inflame the vaginal walls, and by **urinary tract infections (UTIs)**, which can irritate the urethra and bladder. The sexually transmitted diseases **chlamydia** and **gonorrhea** do not themselves cause significant pain in the early stages, but if left untreated, either can progress to a condition known as **pelvic inflammatory disease (PID)**, which can result in lower abdominal pain and dyspareunia. The genital lesions caused by STDs such as herpes may also result in painful intercourse. (We talk at length about STDs in chapter 3; yeast and urinary tract infections are covered in chapter 4.)

Q: You mentioned inadequate lubrication. What would cause this?

A: Sexual arousal will usually release enough natural lubricant so that the vagina is ready for penetration, but a number of factors may alter this process. Apart from the effects of menopause, which shortly we discuss in detail, vaginal dryness can be brought on by breastfeeding, use of superabsorbent tampons and medications such as oral contraceptives, over-the-counter (OTC) cold medications (antihistamines) and antidepressants. Dryness problems often can be solved with use of one of the growing number of lubricants now marketed as aids in lovemaking, such as K-Y Jelly, Astroglide, Aqualube and others.

Equally important is the possibility that insufficient lubrication reflects a lack of arousal. If this is the issue, therapists often recommend both lubricants and a longer period of stimulation before attempting penetration of the vagina.

Q: What are the anatomic problems related to painful intercourse in women?

A: A long list of gynecological disorders may contribute to painful intercourse in women, including **polyps**, **cysts**, **fibroid tumors** and **endometriosis**, the latter a condition in which tissue from the uterus implants on other organs. Another relevant condition is **vaginismus**, which affects 2 to 3 percent of women and causes powerful spasms in the vagina that make penile penetration uncomfortable or impossible. Irritation may also be due to postsurgical scarring or chemicals found in contraceptives or douches.

In general, if you have a chronic problem with pain, it would be advisable to see a medical professional for a thorough evaluation. As you can see from the partial list of causes given here, the roots of dyspareunia can be difficult to diagnose, and too many women are left to believe their conditions are "all in their heads" when they aren't.

Sex and Aging: Hormone Deficiency

Q: There seems to be a lot of controversy about therapy with **estrogen** these days. What is estrogen's basic role in female sexuality?

A: The hormone estrogen is critical to development of the female reproductive system. In response to the signals from the pituitary gland—the body's hormonal control center—a girl begins to secrete estrogen from the ovaries a number of years before **menstruation** begins. From that point on, estrogen is produced on a regular monthly cycle and released from the ovaries.

It has a role in the development of egg follicles and the release of eggs into the **fallopian tubes** (see chapter 5). After the eggs are released, a second hormone called **progesterone**, also produced by the ovaries, signals the beginning of the menstrual cycle.

Some researchers have contended that a woman's periods of peak sexual arousal also correspond to the release of estrogen, but most studies dispute this theory. This monthly cycle of estrogen and progesterone production typically continues until a woman is in her late 40s or early 50s.

Q: What happens then?

A: At some point in her life, a woman will experience a marked change in estrogen production, which leads to menopause—the permanent end to menstruation. Menopause usually takes place between the ages of 45 and 55, although some women experience their last period in their 60s, and others in their 30s. **Ovary** removal, chemotherapy and other circumstances can abruptly bring on menopause.

Menopause is preceded by a time known as **perimenopause**, during which fluctuating estrogen levels cause irregular menstrual periods and, in roughly 15 to 20 percent of women, symptoms such as hot flashes. A hot flash is a physical sensation of intense heat lasting three to six minutes that raises the pulse and often causes a skin flush followed by chills.

After reaching menopause itself, most women do experience some signs and symptoms, though many of these resolve as the body adjusts to its new, lower estrogen level. Up to 90 percent of American women experience hot flashes at some point, but in half of those affected, the flashes stop occurring within a year. In addition, only 20 percent of women experience them for more than two and one-half years. Other potential symptoms include mood swings, insomnia, irritability, weight gain, changes in body shape and changes in the genital tract.

Q: What's the likely impact of menopause on a woman's sex life?

A: First, let us say that it's important to get beyond the stereotype that postmenopausal women no longer enjoy sex. On the negative side, because estrogen is partly responsible for the internal upkeep of the genitals and **urinary tract**, sexual health can be affected. As a woman's estrogen production fades, her vulva and vaginal folds flatten and her vagina may constrict and lose much of its natural lubrication. Vaginal infections, too, may become more frequent. Some 59 percent of women report problems such as vaginal dryness, decreased sexual drive and painful intercourse. For those who experience these symptoms, there are a variety of effective treatments.

Regardless, one survey reports that a surprising 90 percent of postmenopausal women say they are happy with their sex lives— the same proportion that reported sexual satisfaction before menopause. More than 80 percent say that they continue to feel desirable and that they feel more comfortable with their bodies than they did when they were younger. Freedom from contraception and unwanted pregnancy are two factors that play a role in these positive feelings about sex at midlife.

Q: Is it possible to treat menopausal symptoms?

A: It should be said that menopause is a natural process, not a disease. Researchers disagree on how aggressively to use therapy for menopause-related ailments, but both sexual complaints and more general symptoms can be addressed. In many cases, therapy for about two years will get a woman through the period of menopausal symptoms.

Historically, the biggest medical issue surrounding menopause has been the link between falling estrogen levels and increased risk of osteoporosis (brittle bones) and heart disease. It is the concern about these two risks that has driven the trend to place a large number of women on **hormone replacement therapy**.

Q: How does a woman take estrogen?

A: Hormone replacement therapy is basically an attempt to mimic the daily release of estrogen by the ovaries by using pharmaceutical products. There are four major ways of delivering the estrogen:

- *Oral medication.* There are more than half a dozen different formulations of oral estrogen, and one of them, Premarin, is the most frequently prescribed medication in the United States. Oral medication is taken once or twice a day.

- *Transdermal patch.* An adhesive estrogen patch, such as Estraderm or Vivelle, is worn on the buttocks or lower abdomen, releasing estrogen directly into the skin. A patch should be changed twice a week.
- *Vaginal cream.* A measured amount of estrogen cream can be inserted directly into the vagina, an effective approach for vaginal symptoms but not recommended for more severe symptoms or long-term prevention of osteoporosis.
- *Estrogen ring.* This product, known as Estring, is inserted into the vagina, where it releases the hormone slowly over the course of three months. It can be inserted without the help of a health care provider.

Q: But what about progesterone? Doesn't that need replacing, too?

A: Yes. Authorities say that estrogen replacement should be supplemented with doses of progesterone that keep the system in balance. In fact, experts agree that unopposed estrogen—that is, estrogen taken without progesterone—is not recommended for a woman who still has a uterus.

A variety of approaches and doses are used; most are oral medications. Some practitioners will prescribe progesterone replacement for 10 to 14 days out of the month, mimicking the natural cycle before menopause. Others may advocate a small daily dose. Some estrogen formulations are a mix of estrogen and progesterone.

Q: What are the long-term benefits and risks of hormone replacement for women?

A: Estrogen lowers the risk of osteoporosis and reduces the risk of heart disease, the leading killer of older women in the United States. Recent studies suggest that the hormone may also reduce the risk of Alzheimer's disease, improve memory and prevent colon cancer, though further research is needed to confirm these findings.

Despite the beneficial uses of estrogen replacement, some studies have shown it can increase the risk of breast cancer by about 30 percent in women who use it for longer than five years. Experts disagree on the risk, so more specific studies are under way. The Women's Health Initiative, sponsored by the National

Institutes of Health, is testing the effects of hormone therapy on not only breast cancer but also heart disease and osteoporosis.

The leading side effects of hormone replacement are temporary. They include fluid retention, breast tenderness, weight gain and nausea.

Q: Does estrogen replacement lead to better sexual experiences for menopausal women?

A: It can, but other measures can be tried first. Experts on menopause point out that changes such as vaginal dryness occur gradually, and it may be years before they become acute. If the symptoms center on lubrication, a woman can simply use an OTC lubricant such as K-Y Jelly, Astroglide or Aqualube. OTC vaginal moisturizers such as Replens and Gyne-Moistrin may be even more helpful in restoring premenopausal elasticity to the vagina.

These approaches fall short when the problem goes beyond lubrication. Thinning of the vaginal lining and other vaginal changes at menopause may cause discomfort or irritation that may require hormone replacement therapy. Usually the first line of therapy is vaginal cream, which alleviates symptoms such as dryness within a few weeks and often gives greater relief than pills or patches because the effect of the medication is local. Estring, the ring that is inserted into the vagina to release a steady supply of estrogen, is another option. Either Estring or estrogen creams offer a smaller estrogen dose with fewer side effects than pills or patches, an important consideration for women worried about breast cancer. But those who are at higher risk of osteoporosis or heart disease may need the higher dose, so they may decide to choose a systemic method (such as pills or patches) as long as they have no risk factors preventing them from taking hormones.

Q: Are hormones besides estrogen and progesterone used in hormone replacement?

A: Though still controversial, there is growing support for the notion that a lack of testosterone is a cause of diminished sexual drive in postmenopausal women. Accordingly, some physicians have begun recommending that a very small amount of testosterone be added to estrogen and progesterone therapies. This approach has been shown to increase desire in women who have had hysterectomies (and thus have undergone surgical menopause), but the evidence isn't as clear for women going through natural menopause. Plus, the long-term effects are unknown. Possible side effects include increased growth of body hair, oily skin and increased blood pressure.

Q: Are problems of sexual function at menopause a legitimate reason to see a health care professional?

A: Absolutely. We would advise any woman who experiences these symptoms to consult a medical professional about ways to manage the problem. Unfortunately, survey results show that sexual function is not as frequently discussed with health care providers as are other aspects of menopause—partly because of the embarrassment that women may feel in broaching the subject.

PROBLEMS AND CONCERNS FOR MEN

Anorgasmia

Q: What are the causes of anorgasmia in men?

A: First, a caveat: Anorgasmia is not an important clinical issue in men compared with related problems such as **loss of desire**, difficulty achieving or sustaining erections or the tendency to reach climax too quickly—called **premature ejaculation**—all of which we discuss later in this section.

That said, men, too, can have difficulty reaching orgasm. In the National Health and Social Life Survey published in 1994, some 15 percent of men reported having had "difficulty achieving orgasm" in the past 12 months.

Age is an important variable. Older men tend to require more stimulation to achieve an erection and also reach climax less quickly. A higher percentage of older men report the experience of not being able to have an orgasm.

Another major cause of this problem is anxiety about sexual performance, which can delay orgasm or leave a man unable to reach orgasm during a sexual encounter. Anorgasmia also can have physiological causes such as illness or side effects from drugs such as sedatives, which may minimize the sensations needed for climax. Antidepressants may have a similar effect.

Q: Antidepressants seem to be a big concern. Is it true that antidepressants lead to anorgasmia in men?

A: Anorgasmia, strictly speaking, is rarely a side effect of antidepressant drugs in men or women, but the impact of antidepressant drugs on sexual performance is important, particularly the class of mood-altering drugs known as selective serotonin reuptake inhibitors (SSRIs). Recent research on three of the leading SSRIs—fluoxetine (Prozac), sertraline (Zoloft) and paroxetine (Paxil)—showed a four- to eightfold delay in ejaculation compared with the average times for the men taking part in the study. (Their wives literally timed the duration of vaginal intercourse!)

It's important to add that SSRIs don't have the same effect on all men, nor do all SSRIs cause delayed ejaculation: Fluvoxamine (Luvox), for example, was shown to differ from the three SSRIs listed above. In addition, there are other effective antidepressant medications that have minimal or no sexual side effects.

Q: How does delayed ejaculation affect sexual relationships? Is it a problem?

A: The impact of delayed ejaculation on sexual relationships will vary a lot from one couple to the next. In the study cited above, the average baseline time to ejaculation was actually less than one minute, and the delay caused by the SSRIs was not seen as a problem. On the other hand, for those whose baseline time to ejaculation was 10 to 15 minutes, the researchers said, the delay of orgasm induced by some SSRIs might cause some couples simply to give up on intercourse.

Q: What if the problem isn't a medication? Is there a way to treat this type of anorgasmia in men?

A: Yes. The root of the problem is often anxiety about ejaculating; in other words, a man might be capable of reaching the threshold of orgasm but holds back because he is embarrassed or afraid to emit semen. For this problem, the approach taken by therapists is generally to help a man overcome his fear through a series of exercises in which he masturbates first alone, then with a partner. By doing this, a man can become more comfortable with the process and move on to penetrative sex with a partner if he chooses.

Q: When is ejaculation considered to be premature?

A: In essence, premature ejaculation is less a function of time than timing. Ejaculation early in the course of sexual activities is a problem only when it frustrates one or both partners. For this reason, sex therapists today frame the issue broadly as one of "ejaculatory control."

According to Bernie Zilbergeld, Ph.D., author of *The New Male Sexuality*, approximately one-third of all men have difficulty controlling the timing of ejaculation. Usually, the issue for men is reaching climax more quickly than they would like, although as we have seen, delayed ejaculation also can be troublesome. In either case, timing issues can create anxieties for men about performing well and pleasing a partner, which can worsen the problem.

In the case of early ejaculation, sexual partners, for their part, may be reluctant to offer sexual stimulation for fear of creating an early climax or may engage in futile efforts to climax at the same time.

Questions about ejaculatory control are frequently posed by both by men and their female partners, reflecting in part basic differences in male and female sexual response. Men, for example, tend to reach a stage of intense sexual arousal more quickly than women, and men as a rule also find vaginal intercourse a quicker path to orgasm than do women. For this reason, learning to control the timing of ejaculation, at least to some extent, is an important skill in male-female lovemaking.

Q: If a man has a tendency to reach climax quickly, what can he do to break this pattern?

A: Sex therapists report being able to treat ejaculatory problems successfully in up to 90 percent of men by teaching these men a series of exercises. These include cognitive exercises to change one's thinking about orgasm and specific ways of masturbating to discover which sensations are most likely to lead to climax. For example, a man might be instructed to stroke the penis slowly to achieve full erection and then to stop for a minute or change the nature of the stimulation as arousal approaches the point of climax. The aim of these exercises often is to teach men how to recognize a high level of arousal and then to change the nature of the stimulation so that they don't reach the point where ejaculation becomes inevitable.

Q: What about the idea of constricting the head or base of the penis to delay climax? How does this work?

A: The so-called squeeze method is an older approach, developed by Masters and Johnson. With this method, a man or his partner uses the thumb and first two fingers to grasp the penis just below the **glans** (the head) and squeeze for several seconds periodically during sex play. This has the effect of postponing the need to ejaculate, but it must be repeated, especially before vaginal intercourse. A related technique used during vaginal intercourse involves squeezing the base of the penis at intervals during thrusting to delay orgasm. Both methods may require some practice.

Erectile Problems

Q: What is impotence?

A: While the word has many meanings (literally, a "lack of power"), the term has been used in the medical literature to denote a man's inability to get or sustain an erection sufficient for satisfying sex. More recently, clinical researchers have begun to use the more precise terms "erectile difficulty" or **"erectile dysfunction (ED)"** to describe these two conditions.

ED can be a chronic sexual health problem, but it's important to put the term in context. Virtually all men will experience difficulty getting an erection in some circumstances, possibly because of anxiety, fatigue or too much alcohol, for example. If a man does experience a few episodes in which he can't have or keep an erection, it's unwise to spend time worrying about the problem because this can create a psychological barrier to arousal. Remember: Such episodes are normal; they are generally not harbingers of any chronic problem.

Estimates of the number of American men with chronic ED range from roughly 10 million to 18 million. Studies show that half of men over age 40 have at least intermittent problems with ED.

Q: What are the leading causes of ED?

A: The causes of ED break down broadly into three categories: psychological problems, medical conditions and the adverse effects of medication. It was formerly thought that erectile dysfunction was mainly a psychological issue, but more recent data show that the problem is usually physical. In fact, in one Veterans Administration study, only 14 percent of ED cases had psychological causes. Impotence can be a sign or a symptom of a more serious medical condition, so if you're having a chronic problem with ED, it's best to consult a medical professional to get the proper evaluation and treatment.

Q: What medical conditions cause ED?

A: Some of the major culprits are diseases that affect the vascular system. As we discussed earlier in this chapter, increased blood flow to the penis is the mechanism for erection, and an ailment that slows this process will have a direct result on erectile capacity. Heart disease, high blood pressure and hardening of the arteries, therefore, are implicated in ED. Those with heart disease or high blood pressure who smoke have an increased risk. Diabetes is another frequent factor in ED, and this, too, stems from the ill effects of diabetes on blood circulation.

Hormonal problems are another important category. Each day, men secrete quantities of the hormone testosterone, which plays a major role in sexual function. A shortage of this hormone can lead to a loss of interest in sex, to ED and to a longer list of health problems. We talk about all aspects of **testosterone deficiency** later in this chapter.

Other causes of ED include thyroid problems (slow metabolism also slows sexual response); alcoholism and abuse of illegal drugs; spinal cord and other nerve injuries; and problems of the bladder or kidney.

Q: What types of medications contribute to erectile problems?

A: Erectile problems—often temporary, it should be noted—are a possible side effect of a long list of medications, among them the following:

- Diuretics such as bendroflumethiazide (Naturetin), chlorothiazide (Diuril) and spirinolactone (Aldactone)
- Antihypertensives such as propranolol (Inderal), clonidine (Catapres), methyldopa (Aldomet), guanethidine (Isemelin) and Reserpine (Diupres)
- Antidepressants such as clomipramine (Anafranil) and phenelzine (Nardil)
- Antipsychotic drugs such as lithium (Eskalith), fluphenazine (Prolixin) and thioridazine (Mellaril)

The list also includes most types of steroids and most antiepileptic drugs. If you have questions about adverse sexual effects of a medication you're taking, ask your health care provider or pharmacist for details from the product insert, which summarizes the research data.

Q: What about the psychological factors in ED?

A: The leading psychological cause of ED is probably anxiety about performing well sexually. If a man is worried about having or maintaining an erection, he can sometimes fixate on the status of the genitals, and this has the effect of short-circuiting sexual arousal. More generalized stress also can interfere with erections, as can depression. In some cases, there is a fine line between ED per se and more general problems of diminished sexual drive. Depression, which is common among the elderly, may cause loss of desire, but medications used to treat depression can also impair sexual function.

Q: How can you tell which is which?

A: Several tests can be used to sort out physical from psychological causes. The most simple is a blood test to see if testosterone levels are within the normal range. Other procedures include the following:

- *Nocturnal penile tumescence (NPT).* As strange as it may sound, one of the most effective diagnostic tools is to observe the pattern of a man's erections during sleep. Lab technicians attach a painless monitoring device to the penis and then record the frequency and duration of erections during certain phases of sleep. NPT is usually done in a medical school setting or sleep clinic. It's not a perfect test, in part because it assumes healthy sleep patterns even though many people suffer from sleep disturbances. All the same, if the man being monitored produces firm erections when sleeping, the causes of an erectile problem are less likely to be physical than psychological.

- *Measurement of penile firmness by means of a snap gauge or stamp test.* Both of these methods measure nocturnal erections, albeit less scientifically than NPT. The snap gauge is a plastic ring that straps around the penis and is thin enough to break if a full erection occurs. In a homemade version, some people ring the penis with a sealed strip of postage stamps, which, if broken, may show evidence of erections during sleep. The problem with both of these methods is that the gauges may be broken by normal sleep movement. Plus, neither records the number or duration of erections.

- *Injections.* Injections of drugs such as prostaglandin or papaverine will reliably produce erections in men with proper vascular function and offer a good way to confirm that blood supply to the penis is adequate.

Other tests attempt to track blood flow in the penis with ultrasound or x-rays after the injection of a special dye.

While each of these tests has its place, answers are sometimes difficult to come by. ED may have complex causes, perhaps involving both the side effects of medication *and* resulting performance anxiety.

Q: How is ED treated?

A: Up until 1998, only an estimated 10 percent of men with ED actually sought treatment, but that appears to be changing dramatically with the growing array of treatment options. These include the much-heralded oral medication called sildenafil (Viagra). Sildenafil has become one of the fastest-selling prescription drugs of all time since its launch in early 1998. Other treatments, however, can also be quite effective. These include a suppository that is placed in the urethra, penile injection, vacuum pumps, vascular surgery and various prostheses (although most experts agree that prostheses should be viewed as a last resort). The drug **yohimbine**, extracted from an African tree bark, is also available in both over-the-counter and prescription strengths for treatment of ED, though it has been less well studied.

Q: Let's start with Viagra. How does it work?

A: The drug manipulates enzymes in the penis that control the flow of blood *out of* the penis, not into it. Increased blood flow to the penis during sexual arousal begins to engorge the blood vessels and thus creates the conditions for an erection, but erections can't be achieved unless the veins that carry blood back out of the penis become somewhat constricted and keep the blood in place. Taken one hour before sexual activity, Viagra, in essence, temporarily shuts off the exit valves. Thus, if arousal takes place, it won't be physiologically undone. A single dose of the drug will have a measurable effect for roughly eight hours.

In clinical trials, those taking Viagra report a threefold increase in the number of successful attempts at intercourse versus those taking a placebo, or inactive pill. Interestingly, however, female partners give the drug somewhat lower scores.

Q: There have been reports that Viagra can have lethal effects. What's the truth about that?

A: The side effects associated with Viagra are generally mild: headache, indigestion and blurred or tinted vision. Deaths—69 in the first four months the drug was on the market— have been reported among some men taking the medication, but analysis of these cases has yet to show that the drug was at fault. The major caveat—from both the Food and Drug Administration (FDA) and the drug's manufacturer—is that sildenafil is potentially dangerous in men taking nitroglycerin and long-acting nitrates used for heart conditions.

Concerns also have been expressed about the theoretical risk of **priapism** as an adverse effect. Priapism is a condition in which the penis remains erect for several hours, resulting in moderate pain and potential long-term damage. However, this *did not* occur in the first clinical trials of sildenafil.

Q: What about the cost of Viagra? Will health insurance and managed care plans pay for it?

A: At this writing, several of the major insurers were refusing coverage of Viagra, which costs roughly $10 per pill, or else putting in place specific limitations on its coverage, such as a limit to the number of pills allowed per month. Some said that they were conducting reviews of the product's safety before adding it to their formularies.

Q: OK, enough about Viagra. How does the urethral suppository work? What are its relative merits?

A: The urethral suppository, called alprostadil (Muse), comes in the form of a tiny pellet that is inserted through a push-button applicator into the urethra at the tip of the penis. The drug delivers prostaglandin by way of the urethral lining to the soft tissue of the penis. This usually results in a firm erection in five to 10 minutes, though a man whose penile arteries are not functioning properly may not be helped by this approach because the increased blood flow exits the penis too quickly to create tumescence. Erections last 30 to 60 minutes.

At an estimated cost of $18 per dose, the suppository does not require an elaborate apparatus and works well, increasing the frequency of erections in men taking the drug threefold over those taking a placebo in some clinical trials. But many men find that inserting the pellets is painful or causes irritation of the penis, and this method also carries the disadvantage that couples sometimes have to interrupt lovemaking for the medication. This type of therapy is reimbursable by some but not all health insurance plans.

Q: Speaking of painful, why would anyone give himself a shot in the penis?

A: Penile injection, which uses a very fine gauge needle, is reportedly not nearly as painful as it might sound. In fact, most reports of pain with this drug center on the workings of the drug itself. Injection involves combinations of several drugs—among them the active ingredient of the urethral suppositories—which acts on the tissue of the penis and dilates arteries inside the penis to create and prolong erection. Men generally get firm erections 15 to 30 minutes after injection, and the erections last another hour.

At a cost of $18 per dose, this method will reliably produce erections that feel normal. But the necessity of using the needle is a major barrier for many men, and there is also a small chance that the drug will produce local irritation. In a small number of cases, it may also result in priapism, which can cause serious damage if not treated quickly. As with Viagra, the therapy is reimbursable by some but not all health insurance plans.

Q: How does the vacuum pump work? What are its relative merits?

A: With the vacuum pump method, a man places a hollow cylinder over the shaft of his penis and draws out air with a hand pump; the resulting vacuum moves blood into the penis. After the cylinder is removed, a tension ring placed at the base of the penis restricts the outflow of blood. With a one-time investment of $150 to $500, vacuum pumps may be a less expensive option than prescription drugs such as Viagra, but they do have serious drawbacks. For one, they do interrupt lovemaking. Also, the erection produced by a pump is not as rigid as one produced naturally or by some of the methods listed earlier. Finally, pumps may cause irritation of the urethra or abrasion or damage to the penis if the ring at the base of the penis is left in place for more than 30 minutes.

Q: I've heard that the erections created by implants are far different from natural erections. True?

A: Yes. Penile implants come in two varieties. One type, known as nonhydraulic, consists of a pair of silicone implants that run lengthwise along the shaft of the penis, adding length and heft to the penis even in its flaccid state—in essence a permanent erection, but one that is malleable and can be concealed under clothing.

The hydraulic implants are hollow cylinders that can be inflated with a tiny mechanical pumping device that is inserted along with them. Activating these implants sometimes involves manipulating a pump in the scrotum or manipulating the head of the penis to begin the inflation process. The same pump is used to deflate the implants.

In either case, erections are neither as wide nor as long as a natural erection, though they are adequate for vaginal intercourse and can be achieved on demand. A disadvantage of inserts is that they are not reversible. They also change the structure of the penis in ways that render ineffective some of the methods we listed before. Additionally, a problem such as malfunction of the pumping device will require further surgery, which can cost several thousand dollars. For these reasons, it may be best to try other medical solutions before implants.

Q: Is yohimbine a real drug or a bit of folklore?

A: It's a real drug, sold both as a prescription and over the counter. Yohimbine (Yocon, Yohimex and others) is presumed to work by increasing blood flow to the penis and by decreasing the exit of blood. It has a reputation as a complementary medicine, but it has been studied scientifically and approved for the treatment of ED and delayed orgasm. It does have some potentially adverse effects, such as irritability, anxiety and an increase in heart rate and blood pressure. Given the emergence of several other effective therapies in recent years, experts predict its use will probably decrease.

Q: How does aging affect erections?

A: Even in the absence of illness, men undergo a host of physiological changes that alter their sexual appetites and performance—everything from changes in blood flow and hormone levels to the way the nervous system responds to stimuli. A well-documented by-product of this natural aging process is that men require more direct stimulation to get an erection as they get older, and erections tend to become less firm. But these same factors that slow erections may also make it possible for older men to have intercourse for longer periods of time before reaching climax. This change in the nature of erections occurs gradually over time, and it generally *does not* mean that men cannot have erections firm enough for intercourse. Therapists are quick to point out that even a decline in the number of erections doesn't preclude having sex in the broadest sense since older couples are more likely to engage in touching and caressing and to see this as an important part of their sexual relationships.

Sex and Aging: Hormone Deficiency

Q: You mentioned changes in hormone levels as a man ages. What does this have to do with sexual performance?

A: One aspect of male aging is a gradual decline in the male hormone testosterone, and falling levels of this hormone can have a direct impact on sexuality, including the desire for sex and the firmness of erections, as well as on other aspects of a man's health.

Q: How does the body produce testosterone? What does it do, exactly?

A: Almost all of the body's testosterone supply is produced and stored in the testes. It's released into the bloodstream throughout the day, with levels highest in the morning.

As the most important male sex hormone, testosterone plays many different roles over time. At puberty, a surge in the amount of testosterone circulating in the body triggers the development of the mature male body, including increased muscle mass, facial hair, a deepening of the voice and the production of sperm. After puberty, testosterone helps to maintain sexual drive and potency as well as energy, bone density and strength.

Testosterone deficiency occurs when the functioning of the testes is impaired or when there is a defect in the pituitary gland, which stimulates testosterone production.

Q: When does testosterone production begin to wane?

A: Testosterone levels generally begin to fall when men are in their late 40s. To put this in perspective, most men retain sufficient levels of testosterone to maintain sexual activity well into old age. However, about 20 percent of men over age 50 experience a drop in testosterone production that brings their levels well below those of younger men. And when levels fall dramatically, medical complications can result. Aging is the most common cause of testosterone deficiency; other causes include genetic abnormalities, infection or injury to the testes and certain treatments such as chemotherapy and radiation therapy.

Q: What are the signs and symptoms of testosterone deficiency?

A: In older men, physicians may question hormone balance if they see a decline in certain male characteristics, such as a reduction in body hair, muscle mass and sexual drive. One sexual index of testosterone levels is the morning erection: From puberty on, men often awaken from sleep with an erection. But as testosterone levels decline, these erections tend to become less frequent. Also, voluntary erections may be less firm or of shorter duration. The prostate gland may shrink, and the breasts may become enlarged.

Testosterone deficiency may be accompanied by changes such as fatigue or low energy, irritability, loss of motivation and depression. Serious long-term testosterone deficiency may weaken the muscles or lead to osteoporosis, a decrease in bone density that leads to an increased risk of fracture. While osteoporosis is usually associated with women, it can sometimes affect men.

Taken together, the effects of testosterone deficiency would seem to be obvious cause for concern, but in reality the process is a gradual one, and identifying the symptoms hinges on subjective assessments: How much has my erection pattern changed? Am I really more irritable—how much more? Such judgments can be difficult.

Q: How is testosterone deficiency diagnosed?

A: The diagnosis is usually fairly straightforward and is based on a complete medical history and a blood test that measures the total amount of testosterone circulating in the bloodstream. Since levels are higher in the morning, blood is usually drawn early in the day. Men with morning levels below a certain threshold are considered testosterone-deficient.

The decision to treat or not will usually be based on the severity of a man's complaints and his complete medical history.

Q: When and how is it treated?

A: Three types of testosterone replacement therapy are currently available in the United States: oral tablets, intramuscular injections and transdermal delivery systems.

- *Oral medications.* Pills, while easy to use and relatively low in cost, may require multiple doses per day. Over time, they may cause liver damage.
- *Intramuscular injection.* Administered in two- or three-week cycles, injections sometimes create unnaturally high levels of testosterone immediately after treatment and low levels later in the cycle. Men who are sensitive to these peaks and valleys may experience disturbing fluctuations in mood, energy level and sexual function. Also, the injections themselves can leave bruises.
- *Transdermal patch.* This, the newest form of testosterone replacement therapy, delivers consistent amounts of testosterone through a small coin-size adhesive patch, which mimics the normal daily pattern of testosterone production—higher in the morning, lower as the day goes on. One type is worn on the scrotum, replaced every 24 hours; the other requires two patches per day, worn on the upper arms, thighs, back or abdomen.

Q: Does testosterone replacement have risks?

A: Yes. First of all, it is absolutely not recommended for men with normal levels: It will not boost sexual drive and may interfere with the normal process of hormone production. In addition, men weighing therapy should consider that testosterone replacement *may* increase the risk of breast cancer and prostate cancer. There is no definitive finding on these risks, but men who already have breast or prostate cancer are not candidates for therapy, and those who intend to use hormone replacement should first be screened for cancer.

PROBLEMS OF DESIRE

Q: What is meant by loss of desire?

A: Loss of desire—also called loss of **libido**—is actually a catchall term for a complicated set of issues centering on a disinterest in sex or a tendency to spurn sexual activity with a partner. In the medical literature today, the phrase "loss of desire" is used much less frequently than terms such as "low desire" or "desire discrepancy," reflecting the fact that desire issues are more often a matter of degree than a total disinterest. Therapists report that desire problems, rather than specific sexual function problems such as anorgasmia, are perhaps the most frequent reason that couples seek professional help.

Desire problems are sometimes highly individual, reflecting past trauma or deep feelings of inadequacy, for example. Medical conditions such as chronic diseases and depression can also sharply reduce the sexual drive. More commonly, though, desire problems reflect a mismatch in the sexual preferences or emotional needs of a couple.

Q: What are the medical conditions that can lead to low desire?

A: As discussed earlier, hormone imbalances can block desire. So can any number of medications, including treatments for high blood pressure, anxiety, epilepsy, depression and even cancer (chemotherapy). Also, a number of diseases can have a direct impact on sexual drive or can create circumstances that interfere with sexual expression—the psychological burden of having a chronic illness, for example, or the fear of rejection by a partner.

Depression deserves a specific mention here because it is probably the most important illness implicated in low desire. Depression itself has been shown to reduce sexual drive in many people. And the antidepressant drugs used to treat the problem may actually cause—in a sort of catch-22 way—diminished desire and resulting problems of sexual function, such as delayed orgasm for men.

A physician with training in sexual health should take a thorough history in order to evaluate possible medical causes of low desire.

Q: What if the desire problem isn't a medical problem?

A: Here, too, there are numerous common scenarios. Most frequent is the case where a couple is afflicted by a mismatch in sexual desire. One of the partners, for example, is frustrated by wanting to have sex more often than the other. As a consequence, the partner desiring more sex may feel resentment or hurt, while the other may feel pressured or guilty, leading to a vicious circle of emotional withdrawal and increasing isolation.

The solution may sometimes be as simple as better communication: expressing clearly the need for more physical contact or negotiating a compromise in which the partners arrive at a frequency that works for both. Therapists often encourage couples to talk openly about their specific sexual likes and dislikes in an effort to determine whether the problem is less one of frequency than technique—the feeling that sex "isn't fun anymore." There is, of course, also the possibility that mismatched desire results from emotional problems in the relationship that can be addressed only in more comprehensive counseling.

Q: Can aphrodisiacs be used to boost desire, or are they mostly hype?

A: The FDA defines an aphrodisiac as a food, drink, drug, scent or device that claims to increase sexual desire or improve sexual performance. For some scientists, the operative word here is "claims," but others believe there is some empirical evidence to support the various testimonials for aphrodisiacs.

Chocolate's reputation as a food of love, for example, is thought by some researchers to stem from a substance known as phenylethylamine (PEA), which Theresa Crenshaw, M.D., calls "the molecule of love" in her book *The Alchemy of Love and Lust*. PEA, she says, is a natural form of amphetamine that our own system produces in response to various cues, particularly romantic ones. Chocolate, a delicious meal or other sensory treats also are linked with a chemical messenger in the brain known as dopamine, sometimes called the "pleasure chemical."

Of course, even if some of the aphrodisiac lore stems from a placebo effect, that doesn't mean the whole idea is silly. Lovemaking has a complex psychology, and believing that something is sexy may be a big part of the equation. The sharing of an aphrodisiac can act as a kind of communication between partners, sending a signal that the time is right.

Q: **What about alcohol? Some people seem to connect drinking and sex, but I've heard that alcohol interferes with arousal, particularly erections.**

A: Rather than supercharging sex, having a drink (or two) more specifically helps reduce the anxiety that often comes with dating and sex. Alcohol is a central nervous system depressant and relaxes us so we can "let go" and enjoy ourselves. This, in turn, can pique an interest in sex.

As far as the disadvantages of drinking and sex, it's a well-known fact that drinking too much can cause fatigue and make it difficult to keep an erection. Plus, in the research that's been done on condom use and safer sex, it's also been shown that alcohol or recreational drug use hampers one's ability to make good choices.

Q: **What are pheromones? Are they the aphrodisiac of the future?**

A: Pheromones are chemicals secreted by various animals that affect behavior in other members of the species through scent. Although hard data are often ambiguous, some scientists believe that the human species, too, produces pheromones that make men and women more attractive to one another. Winnifred Cutler, Ph.D., who conducted the pioneering research on human sex pheromones and subsequently authored *Love Cycles: The Science of Intimacy,* reports that she has isolated a chemical copy of the formula for the pheromone excreted by a sexually attractive young man or woman. Still controversial, this is a field of ongoing biochemical research.

3 SEXUALLY TRANSMITTED DISEASES

Q: What are sexually transmitted diseases?

A: The names "sexually transmitted disease" or "sexually transmitted infection" may be a lot more straightforward than the old term **"venereal disease,"** but they still bear some explanation. A sexually transmitted disease (STD) is any disease passed from person to person by sexual contact. Sexual contact includes all forms of penetrating intercourse, oral intercourse and a wide range of activities that might be described as sex play or foreplay. Some STDs can be passed through mere skin-to-skin contact, while others require contact with infected body fluids such as blood, semen, saliva, vaginal secretions or stool. A number of STDs can also be passed from mother to child during pregnancy or at birth.

There are more than two dozen different STDs, which can be caused by very different microbes. Many—chlamydia and gonorrhea, to name two of the most common—are caused by bacteria. Some, such as herpes and **human immunodeficiency virus (HIV)** and **acquired immune deficiency syndrome (AIDS)**, are caused by viruses. Still others are caused by parasites and other microorganisms.

Q: Once and for all, is it true that some STDs actually can be spread through contact with things such as toilet seats and hot tubs?

A: STDs can theoretically be spread from person to person by way of an inanimate object or surface such as a tanning bed or a toilet seat, but the statistical hurdles are so high that they make this occurrence very rare. Many of the bacteria and viruses responsible for STDs don't survive long outside the body. In addition, some of them require friction in order to gain entry into the skin or mucous membranes of a new host. Lastly, with reference to toilet seats, you have to remember that the thick skin of the buttocks and thighs is not especially susceptible to infection. The obvious exceptions to this rule are objects used in penetrative sex (for example, sex toys) and needles used for injecting drugs. Towels or other household objects may also be implicated, particularly in the spread of parasites such as lice, which we discuss later in this chapter.

Hot tubs, too, have sometimes been rumored to be a source of STDs. But the chlorine and other disinfectants used in these tubs are generally deadly to STD microbes. As an editorial in the *Journal of the American Medical Association* once put it, the question of whether you can get an STD from a hot tub depends entirely on what you're doing in the tub.

Q: Who is at risk of getting an STD?

A: Anyone. The risk of acquiring an STD has to do with *what you do,* not who you are. Lots of people have the idea that STDs are unusual diseases that affect only a small segment of the population. On the contrary, STDs are among the most widespread kinds of infectious disease, being outranked only by ubiquitous illnesses such as the common cold. As we mentioned earlier, the Institute of Medicine reports that there are an estimated 12 million new cases of sexually transmitted infections every year in the United States. Taking into account the U.S. population as a whole, the odds that a person will contract an STD over the course of a lifetime are one in four.

One reason for these high rates is that human beings give STDs lots of opportunities to spread. Consider this statistic from the World Health Organization: Worldwide, intercourse takes place 42 billion times per year. That works out to 1,300 ejaculations per second.

Q: How would I know if I had an STD?

A: Identifying STDs is not always easy. Given that there are two dozen STDs, it's impossible to include every symptom in a short list, but here are some of the most common ones:

- Sores, blisters, bumps or rashes on or near the genitals
- Painful urination or an unusual discharge with urination

- Abnormal vaginal discharge or discharge with a strong odor
- Bleeding between menstrual periods
- Pain in the lower abdomen or swollen lymph nodes in the groin

One of the big problems in controlling the spread of STDs, however, is that in many people these diseases are often asymptomatic: They *do not* cause symptoms. In addition, several STDs cause symptoms that are quite subtle and hard to recognize. For example, herpes is so mild that 80 percent of those infected don't know they have it. In many cases, the only way to identify an STD is with a diagnostic test. Because people don't realize they have STDs, they don't seek treatment and may continue to spread the diseases to their sexual partners.

Q: Do STDs pose any long-term health risks?

A: Sometimes. While some sexually transmitted diseases may resolve quickly without complications, others play a role in problems such as the development of cervical cancer, liver disease and reproductive tract disorders that can impair a person's ability to have children. Among the most serious consequences of STDs is the risk they pose to infants who are exposed in the womb or at birth. Many of these children may suffer serious mental retardation or life-threatening illness. Lastly, of course, the most lethal STD is **HIV/AIDS**, which is still incurable.

Q: What are the most common STDs?

A: When surveyed, most Americans name HIV/AIDS along with gonorrhea and **syphilis** as the most common STDs, but actually these conditions are not the most widespread. The STDs with the largest number of new cases reported each year are the bacterial infections chlamydia and **trichomoniasis**, both of which are estimated to afflict millions of people annually. Because both of these infections can be cured, however, a large proportion of those infected in a given year will be free of infection by the next year.

By contrast, some of the viral infections, such as herpes and **human papillomavirus (HPV)**, are not curable. They persist for the life of the person infected, so the total number of infected persons grows each year. Current prevalence for both herpes and HPV is estimated in the *tens of millions* in the United States.

We describe all of the leading viral STDs in depth later in the chapter. First, we discuss the bacterial STDs and parasites, starting with two common infections that have similar symptoms and consequences: chlamydia and gonorrhea.

BACTERIAL SEXUALLY TRANSMITTED DISEASES

Chlamydia

Q: I've heard of chlamydia, but I don't know anything about it. What is it?

A: Chlamydia is a unique type of bacterium that attaches itself to healthy cells and draws on these cells for the elements necessary to grow and invade other cells. It does not belong to the group of bacteria that are normally found in the genital tract but is transmitted sexually through contact with secretions such as semen and vaginal fluids.

Chlamydia is found in 3 to 20 percent of men and women, depending on the population sampled. It is most common in women under 25 years of age. In up to 85 percent of women and 40 percent of men, chlamydial infection is asymptomatic—that is, it causes no symptoms. However, even when asymptomatic, chlamydia can result in serious long-term problems, principally damage to the female reproductive organs.

Q: What kind of reproductive damage are we talking about?

A: Chlamydia is mainly implicated in damage to the fallopian tubes. This, in turn, can lead to **infertility** (defined as the inability to conceive after 12 months of trying). And because chlamydia is so common—with an estimated 4 million new cases each year—it's considered one of the leading preventable causes of infertility.

Chlamydia has also been implicated in ectopic pregnancy— a pregnancy in which the fetus implants outside the uterus, usually in the fallopian tube. This is a potentially deadly medical condition that requires emergency care; it's one of the leading causes of maternal death during pregnancy.

Q: When chlamydia is symptomatic, what are we supposed to look for?

A: When symptoms *are* present, they usually include the following:

In women

- Painful urination
- Abnormal vaginal discharge
- Pain in the lower abdomen

In men

- Painful urination or unusual discharge with urination

Q: If chlamydia usually doesn't cause symptoms in men or women, how do people know they have it?

A: Today, we have a number of excellent diagnostic tests that are quite accurate in detecting chlamydial infection, even when a person has no symptoms.

Increasingly, the preferred tests are those that are run on a sample of urine collected first thing in the morning. Chlamydia can also be grown in a **culture** or detected with less expensive tests, such as a smear that is stained and viewed under a microscope. In some cases, a blood test is used to detect evidence of past infection.

The availability of a urine test has created interest in widespread screening for this common but often asymptomatic infection. Urine tests can be used routinely to screen women who come in for an annual exam. Those who test positive can be treated and cured. Routine testing is recommended for all sexually active adolescents, as well as for women between the ages of 20 and 24 who have had more than one sex partner.

Q: How is chlamydia treated?

A: Treatment requires only a short course of antibiotics, taken orally. The treatment regimens recommended by the Centers for Disease Control and Prevention (CDC) include a single-dose option (azithromycin, brand name Zithromax) or an antibiotic that's taken twice daily for seven days (doxycycline hydrochloride, brand names include Doryx, Monodox and Vibramycin). Either regimen will eliminate the infection within seven days in greater than 90 percent of patients. Testing and treating the partners of those who have chlamydia may be necessary to prevent reinfection.

Q: What if I have a chlamydia infection I don't know about? Should I—can I—be tested for this even if the exposure was years ago?

A: Chlamydia can hang around for years if it isn't treated and can cause serious damage even when it's asymptomatic. If you are seeing a doctor about a fertility issue, you should ask whether a chlamydia screening has already been done. If it hasn't, you can ask about getting a blood test that can tell you if you were infected in the past.

Q: Can chlamydia be contracted through oral sex? If so, will the disease show up in the genital area?

A: Chlamydial infection of the mouth and throat can be contracted through oral sex, resulting in a sore throat and other symptoms. But this type of infection will not manifest itself in the genital area unless it is spread to the genitals through sexual contact. In addition, chlamydia in the mouth or throat is much less common than genital infection.

Gonorrhea

Q: I saw an article in the newspaper recently that mentioned gonorrhea as the "leading reportable disease" or something. What's the story?

A: Gonorrhea is actually the number-one infectious disease among those classified as "reportable" by the CDC. If any health care provider diagnoses a case of a reportable disease such as gonorrhea, she must report the case to the local public health authorities. This way, local health departments have accurate numbers to track the spread of gonorrhea in a given community and can take steps to contain it.

There are an estimated 800,000 new cases of gonorrhea every year, about half of which are officially reported. Much like chlamydia, gonorrhea is a bacterial infection that is asymptomatic in up to three-quarters of women, yet it can damage the reproductive system over the long term, leading to infertility and other reproductive tract disorders. In men, the number of asymptomatic carriers is put at less than 5 percent.

Q: How is gonorrhea transmitted?

A: Gonorrhea typically resides in mucous membranes such as the urethra and the vagina and is spread through unprotected intercourse—vaginal, oral or anal.

Q: What are the symptoms of gonorrhea?

A: The word "gonorrhea" comes from the Greek term meaning "flow of seed," referring to the discharge that is often found in those infected. When symptoms *are* present, they include the following:

In women
- Painful urination
- Abnormal vaginal discharge
- Bleeding between menstrual periods
- Pain in the lower abdomen

In men
- Painful urination or unusual discharge with urination

As an oral infection, gonorrhea can cause sore throat. Rectal symptoms may also occur in some cases, but these are relatively uncommon, especially in women.

Q: How is gonorrhea diagnosed?

A: Typically, a health care professional swabs a woman's cervix or a man's urethra. The resulting sample can be tested by means of a culture or examined under a microscope with a stain that picks up evidence of gonorrhea. As with chlamydia, the future probably holds widespread use of urine tests for gonorrhea.

Q: How is gonorrhea treated?

A: Gonorrhea can be cured with antibiotics—though in some cases treatment is complicated by drug-resistant strains of the bacterium. Several single-dose therapies are available, as well as one-week regimens. Today's treatments for gonorrhea cure the disease in more than 95 percent of patients with a single round of therapy. Recommended treatments include a single oral dose of cefixime (Suprax), a single injection of ceftriaxone (Rocephin) or any of several other antibiotics taken orally. People with drug-resistant strains may require several different regimens before a complete cure is possible.

Before the advent of antibiotics, men often went to painful extremes to deal with the ongoing symptoms of chronic infections. Some men, for example, were so distressed by the chronic discharge of gonorrhea that they acquiesced to having their urethras cauterized (burned) in vain attempts to stop it.

Q: It seems like chlamydia and gonorrhea are very similar. Do health care providers have trouble telling them apart?

A: Based on symptoms alone, yes. What's more, the two STDs are often found in the same people. Between 20 and 40 percent of those infected with gonorrhea are also infected with chlamydia. For this reason, it's common practice in many clinics to treat both infections simultaneously. This often means single-dose therapy for gonorrhea, followed by a week of antibiotics for chlamydia.

It's generally true that a person infected with one STD is at greater risk of having another. The reason: Whatever behavior put the person at risk of the first STD may have created an opportunity for another. For this reason, anyone with one STD should be screened for all of them.

Pelvic Inflammatory Disease

Q: What happens if gonorrhea and chlamydia go untreated? What are the complications?

A: In some cases, these two STDs may resolve without treatment. In others, the microbes that cause the infection can work their way into the genital tract and cause serious complications.

In men, the major complication of chlamydia and gonorrhea is a painful testicular disorder called **epididymitis**. In women, a more frequent—and more severe—long-term complication is pelvic inflammatory disease (PID), a catchall term that refers to infection of the fallopian tubes, endometrium and other pelvic structures.

Pelvic inflammatory disease is not an STD per se but a complication of various types of infections. However, STDs are its leading cause. In the United States, there are an estimated 1 million new cases of PID each year, with up to 80 percent caused by sexually transmitted microbes, depending on the group of people studied. The other 20 percent are brought about by a wide range of infectious agents, including some of the types of bacteria found normally in the vagina. Some studies suggest that douching may play role in spreading these bacteria to the upper genital tract.

Q: What are the symptoms of PID?

A: Like the infections that cause it, PID can sometimes be very subtle and go unrecognized. A common sign of persistent chlamydia or gonorrhea is inflammation of the cervix, which produces the abnormal discharge we referred to earlier. As infection spreads up the reproductive tract, it begins to affect the fallopian tubes or the endometrium, sometimes causing the following symptoms in women:
- Fever (sometimes quite high)
- Severe pain in the lower abdomen
- Irregular vaginal bleeding
- Painful urination and painful intercourse

Q: How is PID treated?

A: Many cases of PID, especially those caused by STDs, are successfully treated with antibiotics. However, prolonged untreated infection can severely inflame the fallopian tubes and create scarring or thin, fibrous growths, called adhesions, that cling to the ovaries or other organs, thus restricting the natural movement of the tubes. This constriction is thought to be partly responsible for the high incidence of infertility and ectopic pregnancy found in women with a history of PID.

Syphilis

Q: No one says much about syphilis anymore. Has it been eradicated?

A: Not completely. This STD was once quite a scourge. Historically, it is perhaps the most important STD. In the late fifteenth century, syphilis spread throughout a Europe torn by war and became known as the "great pox." Even in the first half of the twentieth century, it remained a vexsome infection, afflicting between 5 and 10 percent of the adult population. In fact, it defied fully effective treatment until the late 1940s, when penicillin was first developed.

Because of the effectiveness of modern antibiotics and because of public health efforts to stop its spread, syphilis is now on the decline. The CDC says the number of new cases has plummeted by 84 percent since 1990. Syphilis is now one of the least common STDs in most parts of the United States, though it is still found in select populations and is even considered epidemic in some rural parts of the Southeast.

Q: How is syphilis transmitted?

A: The disease is transmitted through direct contact with a syphilis sore, called a **chancre**, during vaginal, oral or anal sex. The chancre is a single, firm, round, usually painless sore, appearing on the external genitalia, vagina, **rectum**, anus, mouth or lips.

Q: Is a chancre the only symptom of syphilis?

A: No. The chancre develops approximately three weeks after exposure to the microbe and persists for one to five weeks. The appearance of the sore marks the first of three phases associated with syphilis.

The second stage, lasting two to six weeks, begins with the disappearance of the chancre. It is generally characterized by a skin rash that appears at various sites. These rashes include rough "copper penny spots" on the palm of the hand and the bottom of the foot; a prickly heat rash; moist warts in the groin area; and white patches on the inside of the mouth. Fever, swollen lymph glands, headaches and weight loss often accompany the rashes.

Symptoms gradually fade as the virus enters into the third phase, the latent stage, during which serious internal damage begins. If left untreated, syphilis can result in heart disease, arthritis, brain damage, paralysis, blindness, dementia, impotency and even death.

Q: How is syphilis diagnosed?

A: Diagnosis of syphilis in its early stages is usually made by swabbing a chancre and examining the sample under a microscope, a procedure done quickly in the clinic while the sample is fresh. Also available are blood tests capable of detecting syphilis at later stages of the disease.

Q: How is syphilis treated?

A: Fortunately, treatment of this particular STD is also quite simple and inexpensive. One dose of the antibiotic penicillin is usually sufficient for an individual infected for less than a year. For a person infected longer, several doses are necessary. Anyone treated for syphilis should receive a blood test six months and 12 months later to confirm that the syphilis is cured.

Vaginitis

Q: Is vaginitis an STD?

A: Sometimes yes, sometimes no. Vaginitis is an inflammation of the vaginal tissue often accompanied by itching, discharge or a fishy odor. It can be caused by a number of different microbes, some of which can be—but are not always—sexually transmitted. The most common causes of vaginitis are trichomoniasis infection, yeast infection and a bacterial infection known as **bacterial vaginosis (BV)**. Yeast infections really are not STDs, and BV is only sometimes caused by sexually acquired microbes. (We cover both of these in more detail in chapter 4.) Trichomoniasis, however, is indeed an STD.

PROTOZOA: TRICHOMONIASIS

Q: What is trichomoniasis?

A: Trichomoniasis is a common infection caused by *Trichomonas vaginalis,* a type of microbe called a protozoan. It is spread through sexual intercourse and attaches to mucous membranes such as the walls of the vagina or urethra. Even without treatment, it generally resolves in a short period of time and is seldom implicated in long-term complications such as PID.

Q: What are the symptoms of trichomoniasis?

A: Sometimes asymptomatic like other STDs, trichomoniasis causes symptoms in more than half of infected women and less than half of infected men.

When symptoms are present, they include the following:

In women
- Grayish or greenish vaginal discharge, often with odor
- Vaginal itching
- Painful intercourse

- Painful urination (less frequent)

In men
- Irritation of the urethra and cloudy discharge
- Painful urination

Q: How is trichomoniasis diagnosed and treated?

A: Generally, a clinician uses a swab to take a sample of vaginal or urethral discharge. This sample is then placed on a slide and prepared for immediate inspection under a microscope, where trichomonas is easily identified. It can be treated with a single dose of the antibiotic metronidazole (brand names include Flagyl, Metizol and Protostat), but a weeklong course of therapy gives a slightly higher cure rate, especially for infected men. As with all STDs, sexual partners should also be treated.

PARASITES: SCABIES AND PUBIC LICE

Q: Are scabies and pubic lice the same thing?

A: No, but they have several things in common. Both are parasites that infect the skin and are spread through close physical contact, though not exclusively sexual contact. An example would be the sharing of bedclothes or towels. Both parasites cause itching, and both are treated with topical drugs that essentially poison them.

Scabies is an infection caused by the itch mite, a sort of microscopic tick that burrows into the skin and lays eggs, which then hatch and develop into adults within 10 days. Symptoms include itchy lesions on the hands and wrists in a majority of cases. These lesions can also be found on the chest, buttocks, thighs and penis. Scabies is seldom found on the neck or face.

Lice, on the other hand, come in three species that infect humans—head, body and pubic lice. All three are visible to the naked eye and lay eggs (nits) that are visible, usually at the base of hair follicles. As you might guess, pubic lice (also called crabs) are the species most likely to be sexually transmitted.

Q: How is scabies diagnosed and treated?

A: For diagnosis, a health care provider will take a sample of the burrows and examine it under a microscope for the characteristic wavy shape of the burrow. Treatment consists of applying a topical medication—usually permethrin (Elimite, Nix) or lindane (Kildane, Scabene)—over the entire body from the neck down. The ointment is washed off after eight to 12 hours. Antihistamines may be used to quell the itching that sometimes continues after treatment. Frequently, the infected person's family members, who are at high risk of exposure, are also treated, even if they have no symptoms.

Q: How are lice diagnosed and treated?

A: Pubic lice usually are identified based on a medical history and physical examination of either the lice or nits. They can be treated with a variety of topical drugs and shampoo preparations that are applied to the skin and hair and then washed off after a few minutes. Some of the medications used for scabies are also used for lice, including permethrin and lindane. Be careful to follow your health care provider's instructions about which type of formulation to use and how to apply it.

Q: What about infestation in the household? How do you get rid of the lice and scabies that may not be killed by medication?

A: The house does not have to be fumigated, but bedding and clothing should be decontaminated. Wash items in hot water or send them to be dry-cleaned. Lice and crabs will generally die if deprived of a human host for three days.

VIRAL SEXUALLY TRANSMITTED DISEASES

Genital Herpes

Q: What is genital herpes?

A: Genital herpes is an infection caused by **herpes simplex virus (HSV)**, a widespread virus that has two types, HSV-1 and HSV-2. HSV-1 is most often the cause of the sores around the lips or nose that are known as cold sores or fever blisters. HSV-2, which is quite similar in most ways, tends to cause similar symptoms in the genital area.

Q: We don't hear much about herpes anymore. Is genital herpes still widespread?

A: Very much so. Herpes was well publicized in the early 1980s but was overshadowed by the HIV/AIDS epidemic. However, for a variety of reasons that we explain in the next few pages, genital herpes has continued to spread through the sexually active population at alarming rates. At the start of the 1980s, genital herpes was found in approximately 16 percent of adults in the United States, according to the National Health and Nutrition Examination Survey sponsored by the federal government. But by the start of the 1990s, that percentage had increased to 22 percent, translating to 43 million people. Today, it's probably higher.

Q: How could an infection be so widespread and yet so little talked about?

A: For one thing, HSV, the virus that causes herpes, persists in the body for life. Herpes can be treated, but it can't be cured, so the number of persons infected is always increasing. Equally important, herpes is often a very mild infection and goes unrecognized by those who have it. Thus, there are tens of millions of people who are "carriers." An astounding 80 percent of those who carry genital HSV don't realize they have the infection, but they are nonetheless capable of infecting others.

Q: Doesn't herpes cause rather unmistakable symptoms?

A: Sometimes. The so-called classic symptoms of genital herpes would be hard to ignore, particularly during what is called a primary episode, the symptomatic period that sometimes follows a first-time infection. But we have learned in the last 10 years that these "classic" symptoms are not typical. The majority of people with herpes are either asymptomatic or have very subtle symptoms that they fail to recognize as herpes.

Q: What are the classic herpes symptoms?

A: The classic symptoms most often seen in a primary infection include a short period of itching, burning, tenderness and redness on the genitals. **Vesicles** (clear, dome-shaped blisters) may then appear, typically on both sides of the penis or vulva. These vesicles may also be found on neighboring areas, including the thighs, buttocks and anal region. Vesicles on soft, moist external tissues such as the labia minora tend to rupture soon after they appear, leaving painful ulcers (shallow, open sores) that are covered with puslike fluid and surrounded by a distinct halo of reddened skin. On drier surfaces such as the skin of the thighs and buttocks, vesicles tend to remain intact, fill with pus and then dry out, leaving a crust or scab. In a primary episode, the entire process of lesion formation and healing takes about two to three weeks.

Up to 40 percent of men and 70 percent of women also have systemic, flulike symptoms during a primary episode. These include fever, headache, malaise (a vague feeling of bodily discomfort), muscle aches and loss of appetite. Some will also have painful swollen lymph nodes in the groin and pelvic areas.

Q: What happens after a primary episode?

A: Whether a person gets treatment or not, the symptoms of a primary episode will clear up, but HSV remains in the nerve roots, called ganglia, where it sets up a permanent base of operations. From time to time, the virus will reactivate and travel back to the surface of the skin in the genital area or the mucous membranes such as the vagina and anus. These recurrences, also called outbreaks, sometimes appear on the thighs and buttocks.

Recurrent symptoms sometimes mimic the kind of classic herpes described earlier, but symptoms are usually fewer, less painful and don't last as long. Alternately, reactivation may lead to very subtle symptoms such as a reddened area of skin in the genital area, a small lesion resembling a pimple or ingrown hair, or a rash resembling jock itch. Recurrences may last a week or more, but many of them will heal in a matter of days.

Q: Why does herpes recur instead of just going away?

A: The genius of HSV is its ability to hide in the nerve ganglia, where it cannot be reached by antiviral drugs or by the body's immune defenses. Normally, in the course of defending against invaders, the immune system will damage cells in the area of the body it is attempting to protect. This damage is usually temporary because most types of tissue, such as skin or bone, can repair themselves. Nerve cells, however, cannot regenerate or repair themselves. For this reason, immune responses do not reach into the immune system and herpes is able to recur.

Q: Why do so few people with genital herpes have symptoms?

A: It appears to be largely a question of immunity. Some people have better natural defenses against HSV infection. However, what may be a more accurate way of framing the question is to say that most people with genital herpes don't have *recognizable* symptoms. The public has been told for many years that genital herpes always produces severe symptoms. As a result, people with subtle symptoms usually don't think to ask themselves, "Could this be herpes?" It has been shown that when people with supposedly asymptomatic herpes are trained to recognize the subtler symptoms of disease, many are able to identify when they are having an outbreak.

Q: How is herpes diagnosed?

A: Because its symptoms are sometimes subtle, herpes is often difficult to diagnose. Several types of tests are used.
The standard laboratory test is a culture. A health care provider swabs a suspected herpes lesion and sends the sample off to a laboratory. There it is placed in a collection of cells that resemble skin cells and observed for several days. If the sample replicates and spreads, a technician views it under a microscope to see if it is indeed HSV. A second test can be run along with a culture to see if the sample is HSV-1 or HSV-2.

Antigen detection tests are sometimes used instead of a culture. Like a culture, this type of test requires a sample from an active lesion, which is then sent off to a lab for analysis. The antigen test is nearly as accurate as a culture, and results are available more quickly. However, the test does not indicate which type of HSV is present.

The problem with both culture and antigen tests is that getting an adequate sample requires seeing a patient when lesions are still emitting (or "shedding") the virus. Unfortunately, it turns out that if a person with herpes waits even a day or two before seeing a health care provider, the sample may give a false-negative result—that is, the test may indicate that the person does not have herpes when he actually does. For this reason, an important emerging technology in herpes diagnosis is the blood test.

Q: What are the advantages of a blood test?

A: A blood test picks up evidence that the immune system has begun to attack HSV by producing antibodies, substances released into the bloodstream to combat specific invaders, including microbes such as HSV. The presence of these antibodies confirms that a person is infected. The advantage of this method over tests that swab a suspected herpes lesion is that antibodies can be detected at *any time;* the patient doesn't have to come to the clinic with an active lesion. Another advantage is that the latest blood tests can tell which type of HSV is present, HSV-1 or HSV-2.

The disadvantage of the blood test is that it can take a few weeks before the immune system produces sufficient numbers of antibodies to be detected, so it's not necessarily the test of choice for a first-time infection. Also, even if the test is positive, it's not absolute evidence that a current symptom is caused by herpes because the blood test doesn't distinguish between past infection and present infection. In other words, you may have herpes, but it could be another condition that is triggering your current problems.

Q: If you have genital herpes, is it useful to know whether the cause is HSV-1 or HSV-2?

A: It can be useful. Genital herpes caused by HSV-1 is actually less likely to recur, which may be good news if you've been recently diagnosed. It's also sometimes useful to know which type or types you have because it may help you know whether your partner is at risk. If both you and your partner have HSV-1, for example, there is little risk of transmission.

The problem is that there are also some blood tests on the market that are not reliable when it comes to identifying the type of HSV. Ask your health care provider for a Western blot serology for HSV, which is the most accurate test, or call the Health Advice Company at 888-ADVICE-8 for information about new diagnostic kits on the commercial market.

Q: Are any new tests being developed?

A: A new generation of tests coming onto the market will enable health care providers to detect the presence of antibodies to HSV-2 in the bloodstream, based on a sample as small as one collected by a finger prick. These tests should be on the market within two years.

Q: How is herpes treated?

A: There are now three effective treatments for genital herpes—acyclovir (Zovirax), famciclovir (Famvir) and valacyclovir (Valtrex). These drugs seek out herpes-infected cells and cripple the virus's ability to make new copies of itself. (The immune system, of course, also has its own natural defenses against herpes.) Although these drugs can relieve many of the symptoms of genital herpes, they cannot cure it.

Q: If herpes can't be cured, what good does treatment do?

A: Millions of people are routinely prescribed acyclovir or another antiviral herpes drug to lessen the discomfort of their first episodes of herpes. Medication can be used in a similar way to treat—essentially, to shorten—subsequent outbreaks. Since many outbreaks last only a few days, however, getting benefit from treatment requires starting therapy at the first sign of symptoms, such as the itching or tingling feeling that can precede herpes sores. One approach is to get your health care provider to write a refillable prescription for this episode-by-episode therapy so that you can have a supply on hand to initiate treatment without delay. Another option is to obtain a prescription for the relatively new herpes drug valacyclovir, which has been shown to stop roughly 30 percent of outbreaks if taken when symptoms first appear.

For those who have frequent or especially troublesome outbreaks, it may be wiser to consider suppressive antiviral therapy. This involves taking a small amount of an antiviral drug every day in the hope of stopping outbreaks altogether. In large studies, suppressive therapy has lowered the frequency of herpes recurrences by 80 percent.

Q: If people don't have herpes symptoms, are they contagious?

A: What most of us learned about herpes 10 or 15 years ago was that the infection could be spread only when its characteristic sores were present. In between these recurrences, the virus was believed to be completely asleep. Research has since shown that this isn't true: Without causing outbreaks per se, HSV can reactivate and travel the nerve pathways, leaving sufficient quantities of the virus on the skin or mucous membranes to create the risk of transmission. These periods of activity are called by various names in the scientific literature—asymptomatic shedding or subclinical shedding, to be specific—but the key fact about them is that they can result in transmission of herpes from one person to another. In fact, careful studies have shown that more than two-thirds of new herpes cases result from one of these episodes of asymptomatic shedding.

Q: If herpes can be transmitted at virtually any time, what can a person do to keep from infecting a sexual partner?

A: Historically, the major approach to prevention has been to promote abstinence when symptoms are present and condom use at all other times. Condoms are considered effective as all-around STD prevention, but it's known that they can't give complete protection against herpes because herpes sores can appear in places not covered or protected by condoms.

In addition, we now believe suppressive therapy may lower the risk of transmission. We've known for some time that suppressive therapy—taking an antiherpes drug every day—drastically reduces the frequency of symptoms. There is now some evidence that daily therapy also reduces the activity of the virus in between outbreaks, cutting the rate of asymptomatic shedding by as much as 95 percent. Logically, we expect this type of therapy to have a major impact on lessening the risk of transmission, and studies are under way to confirm this hypothesis.

Q: What if a person is diagnosed with genital herpes when he has been in an exclusive relationship for years? Does this mean the person's partner has been fooling around?

A: The sudden appearance of genital herpes in a presumably monogamous relationship does not necessarily mean one partner has been unfaithful.

How one gets genital herpes is a relatively easy question to answer. Genital herpes is transmitted during sexual intercourse (vaginal or anal) and during oral sex. *When* one gets genital herpes is another question altogether. As we noted earlier, up to 80 percent of genital HSV infections produce no recognized symptoms, yet these silently recurring infections are fully capable of delivering infectious virus to genital surfaces. Thus, it is possible for a person to acquire infection when a partner is shedding the virus asymptomatically.

Another scenario that occurs frequently is this: A person will seek medical care for what she thinks is a new infection in the genital area, but diagnostic tests show that it is actually a recurrence of an old infection. Herpes simplex virus can lie low, undetected for years—even decades. Then, for reasons we don't understand, it can begin producing symptoms. In general, if these symptoms are quite severe, the odds are that the infection is primary. If they are mild, one would suspect a recurrence.

Q: Are cold sores around the lips or nose a form of herpes? Can you spread herpes from the mouth or face by kissing?

A: Yes to both questions. The virus associated with cold sores is indeed a herpes simplex virus—usually HSV-1; as we explained earlier, most genital herpes is caused by HSV-2. The two viruses are distinct but very closely related. Actually, the majority of people already have been exposed to and infected with HSV-1 by the time they reach adolescence. Most of them, however, don't have recurring cold sores; rather, they had a bout with herpes in their early years and have since forgotten all about it.

If you have an HSV-1 infection and the person you are kissing is one of the more than 50 percent of Americans who is also infected, that person has immunity to the virus and in all likelihood will not be reinfected. If the person has *not* been infected before, you could pass on HSV-1 herpes through kissing. This could result in an episode of cold sores and possibly recurrent cold sores.

The best advice is to avoid kissing when you have a cold sore—your most contagious period. It's also theoretically possible to transmit HSV-1 during asymptomatic periods, but given the usually benign nature of this common infection, no one seriously recommends that you stop kissing altogether.

Q: What about oral sex? If you have cold sores and have oral sex, can your partner get genital herpes?

A: Yes. HSV-1 can be spread to the genitals during oral sex. That's why between 10 and 50 percent of new genital herpes cases are caused by HSV-1.

Q: Do experts feel that diet and supplements—lysine, for example—can help stop herpes outbreaks?

A: The problem with alternative approaches to herpes is that they are not, for the most part, studied in a scientific way. Some people say that giving up coffee stopped their herpes outbreaks; others say that large doses of vitamin C helped. The list of reported home remedies is endless. But what "works" is highly subjective, and what works for one may not work for all.

Lysine has actually been looked at by researchers. This amino acid was studied by the National Institutes of Health and was shown to have no significant effect in lessening herpes outbreaks.

Generally speaking, if you eat a balanced diet, get adequate sleep and exercise regularly, this healthy lifestyle should result in a better functioning immune system, which in turn should have a positive effect on herpes. But if you are suffering from frequent outbreaks and want to alter the pattern, antiviral medication is the most direct route to alleviating symptoms.

Genital Warts

Q: Are genital warts the same thing as herpes?

A: No. Genital warts are caused by a different virus. Herpes is caused by herpes simplex virus; warts are caused by human papillomavirus (HPV). The two viruses have several things in common: They are transmitted by skin-to-skin contact, are generally benign and often silent and persist for long periods in the body. Tens of millions of Americans—both men and women—have acquired one or both of these viruses through sexual activity.

Q: What do genital warts look like?

A: Genital warts can take a variety of forms. Some are fleshy, cauliflowerlike growths; others are smaller or more subtle—sometimes little more than a bump. Except for large warts aggravated by friction, genital warts generally do not cause pain, itching, bleeding or other symptoms.

Warts can appear in various locations, including the penis and scrotum in men and the vulva in women. Warts in men and women can also appear in the area around the anus.

Q: How are genital warts diagnosed?

A: A health care provider is usually able to diagnose genital warts based on a physical exam and medical history. In some cases, the health care provider may use clinical aids such as strong light or magnification. He may also apply a vinegar solution or a stain to the affected area in an effort to make small warts more visible. Lastly, in some cases, your provider may perform a biopsy. This is an in-office procedure in which the provider removes a small piece of the wart and sends it to a laboratory for further analysis.

Q: What can be done for genital warts?

A: Genital warts can be removed in several different ways. The newest therapies are prescription topical medications (podofilox, brand name Condylox; imiquimod, brand name Aldara) that the patient can apply to the surface of the warts and then wash off later. With these treatments, it may take from four to 16 weeks to clear the warts, depending on the type of treatment and the extent of the warts.

People with genital warts have other options. In-office procedures include the following:

- Freezing the warts (cryotherapy)
- Applying caustic chemicals such as bichloracetic acid
- Removing them surgically

No single method of treating warts has been shown to work best for everyone, and in many cases, multiple treatments are necessary in order to clear warts. In general, it's probably advisable to try the less invasive, patient-applied therapies first and move on to more complex therapies later if topical remedies are unsuccessful.

Q: Does treatment kill HPV altogether?

A: All of the therapies listed here are capable of clearing genital warts, though none is guaranteed to completely eliminate the human papillomavirus from the body. In many cases, genital warts recur, requiring repeat treatment.

Q: Is HPV the cause of cervical cancer?

A: Yes and no. There are more than 70 subtypes of HPV. To put this in perspective, the types of HPV that cause external genital warts—notably type 6 and type 11—are almost never implicated in cervical disease; they are not precursors to cancer. Hence, they are called low-risk types.

On the other hand, there are more than a dozen types of HPV that attack the cervix and significantly increase the risk of cervical disease. These high-risk types, notably types 16 and 18, are thought to work in combination with other risk factors to promote abnormal cell growth. Even when high-risk types are present in the cervix, however, they usually are cleared by the immune system before they result in any real harm.

Q: So if a woman has had genital warts, she doesn't need to worry?

A: She should take some precautions. Any woman with a history of any sexually transmitted disease, such as genital warts, should have regular Pap smears, which are an excellent way to detect potential cervical problems. This test takes a sample of cells from the cervix and examines them for signs of abnormal growth. A woman who has had genital warts should talk with her health care provider about how frequently she should have a Pap smear.

Q: What happens if the Pap smear turns out to be abnormal?

A: When following up an abnormal Pap smear, the health care provider may seek additional information through one or several further tests:

- A repeat Pap smear may be recommended in cases where the abnormality is of unknown significance.
- A colposcope, which is inserted into the vagina, allows a physician to get a magnified view of the cervix and visually inspect abnormal tissue.
- A biopsy takes a sample of the abnormal tissue that can be sent to a laboratory for closer examination.

- HPV typing tests can be run on Pap smears or biopsy specimens. These tests can determine whether the HPV found in the cervix is one of the types linked with risk of cervical cancer.

Q: Do the high-risk HPV types infect men? Do they cause cancer in men?

A: Men undoubtedly can be infected with high-risk types and can spread them to their sexual partners. While less is known about high-risk HPV types in men than women, there is a growing body of research that suggests the high-risk HPV types cause anal and penile cancers in men. These cancers, however, are rare by comparison with cervical disease.

The highest risk of HPV-related cancer in men is seen in those who practice receptive anal intercourse. Some researchers now advocate that high-risk men have the equivalent of a yearly Pap smear on the interior of the anus.

Q: How can I get a specific test for HPV?

A: Typing tests are not done routinely in most clinics, but there are clinics that do them. Currently, the most widely available HPV typing test is called Hybrid Capture. In effect, this test is practical only for women because it is done along with a Pap smear. It can be run directly on a Pap sample collected with the ThinPrep system developed by CyTyc Corporation. It can also be run on cervical biopsy samples.

Q: If a woman has HPV on her cervix, what will the treatment be?

A: Treatment for cervical HPV infection requires a physician with expertise in this area. In general, the goal of treatment is to surgically remove all of the abnormal cervical tissue. The most widely used surgical methods today include laser, scalpel and a form of electrosurgery called loop electrosurgical excision procedure (LEEP). With any of these methods, the abnormal portions of the cervix can be successfully removed in more than 80 percent of patients. Surgery often requires anesthesia but is frequently performed on an outpatient basis, so no overnight hospital stay is involved.

After the affected tissue is removed, patients typically require several weeks to heal fully. In a small number of cases, cervical lesions recur, requiring repeat surgery. Most likely, though, a woman will simply be monitored with more frequent Pap smears to ensure that the treatment was successful.

Q: If HPV is so widespread, how can I avoid getting it?

A: We review the issue of STD prevention in detail later in this chapter, but because HPV is so tough to detect and to stop, we mention the most important precautions here as well.

First, it's known that the risk of acquiring HPV increases with the number of sexual partners you've had in your life, and the same is also true of your partner. That is, if your partner has a large number of prior lovers, your risk increases as well.

Second, it's thought that condoms—used consistently and correctly—may offer some protection against the spread of genital HPV. Condoms offer the best protection against STDs in general, though in one study they showed no benefit in preventing HPV.

Third, if you or a partner has a genital wart or a cervical lesion, consider that site to be a source of infectious virus until it's removed. So refrain from sexual activities that involve contact with that lesion. You should also stop smoking and make sure you eat a balanced diet, because nutritional deficiencies—of folic acid, for example—are linked with increased risk of cervical disease.

Hepatitis

Q: Is hepatitis a sexually transmitted disease?

A: Sometimes. Hepatitis is defined as an inflammation of the liver, but it is often the result of viral infections that are sexually transmitted. Hepatitis B virus (HBV) is the most prevalent form of viral hepatitis. Spread readily through contaminated blood, HBV can be transmitted in blood transfusions and is found in significant numbers of people who share needles to inject illegal drugs.

HBV is also found in other body fluids such as semen, vaginal secretions, stool and even saliva. Sexual contact accounts for 30 to 60 percent of the new HBV infections each year in the United States.

Q: What are the symptoms of hepatitis B infection? How is it diagnosed?

A: First, like many STDs, HBV can strike silently. Some people carry the virus without knowing it. Others develop symptoms, including the following:

- Jaundice (a yellowing of the skin and eyes)
- Nausea, fatigue and other symptoms associated with a gastrointestinal virus
- Dark urine

It is diagnosed through a blood test that detects specific antibodies to HBV.

Q: How is hepatitis B infection treated?

A: For cases of severe hepatitis, a number of therapies are under study, including medications using interferon, a substance produced by the body to combat viral infection.

People exposed to blood, semen or other fluids likely to be infected with HBV are treated as quickly as possible through injections of an immune-boosting agent called hepatitis B immune globulin. The object of this treatment is to prevent HBV from reproducing (also called replicating) and causing disease. These individuals are also given the HBV vaccine in order to build protection against further exposure.

Q: Is the hepatitis vaccine safe?

A: Yes. Several vaccine manufacturers have marketed vaccines that do not use live virus. These vaccines are now recommended for all newborns, for 11- and 12-year-olds who have not yet been vaccinated and for adults in high-risk groups, such as those with multiple sex partners and those who inject illegal drugs. Vaccination consists of a series of shots: an initial vaccination followed by two booster shots at intervals of one to two and four to six months. This series is presumed to confer lifelong protection.

HIV/AIDS

Q: What is HIV? How does it differ from AIDS?

A: HIV stands for human immunodeficiency virus; AIDS is the acronym for acquired immune deficiency syndrome. The two terms are often used synonymously, but they should not be confused.

Like several other viruses listed in this chapter, HIV persists in the body for a long period of time. Unlike a herpes virus or a wart virus, however, HIV directly attacks the immune system, rendering it ineffective against other infections. This assault on the immune system may not immediately cause disease, but after a while, the immune system usually weakens. If it does, even commonplace infections that resolve quickly in a person with normal health are capable of causing serious illness. An HIV-infected person is clinically diagnosed with AIDS when she suffers a major deterioration of immune function or begins to have bouts with one of several different illnesses.

Q: How is HIV transmitted?

A: It's spread through the blood, semen or vaginal secretions of an HIV-infected person. People can get HIV infection when they have contact with these fluids. The most likely causes of this exposure are sexual intercourse or the injection of illegal drugs with shared needles. In addition, HIV-infected women can pass the virus to their newborns during pregnancy and childbirth.

Q: I've heard that people can get AIDS from blood transfusions? Is this true?

A: Some people who received blood products before March 1985 received HIV-infected blood because HIV screening was not yet in standard practice. Today, all donated blood is being screened for HIV.

Q: What about getting HIV from casual contact—beverage glasses, doorknobs, that sort of thing?

A: Although small amounts of HIV have been found in body fluids such as saliva, feces, urine and tears, there is no evidence that HIV can be transmitted through these body fluids. By studying the families of those who have HIV infection, researchers have determined that the virus is not spread through casual contact such as the sharing of food utensils, towels, telephones or toilet seats.

Q: What are the early symptoms of HIV?

A: The symptoms are quite varied. For four to seven weeks after a person is infected with HIV, the virus replicates and spreads at a fast rate. In 30 to 60 percent of infected individuals, this causes flulike symptoms such as the following:
- Fever
- Swollen lymph nodes in the neck and groin
- Headache
- Malaise

Q: What happens then?

A: These symptoms often resolve and usually usher in a period of asymptomatic infection, though lymph nodes often remain swollen.

Unfortunately, HIV continues to multiply during this time and eventually can overwhelm the immune system. At this point, common infections such as herpes that are usually mild in a person with a healthy immune system can cause serious illness in the person with HIV. In the medical literature on HIV, these common infections are known as "opportunistic infections."

Q: What sorts of common infections are we talking about?

A: Opportunistic infections include problems such as recurrent yeast infections, severe outbreaks of oral or genital herpes, forms of pneumonia and several others.

Q: How is HIV diagnosed?

A: HIV can be diagnosed by a blood test even in its asymptomatic periods. Currently, the two most common tests are the enzyme-linked immunosorbent assay (ELISA) and the Western blot test, both of which look for antibodies to HIV. Some of the newer tests look for antibodies in a sample of fluid from inside the mouth.

As with herpes, however, it may take the immune system several weeks to manufacture these antibodies; therefore, neither of these tests can be accurately performed until after the HIV "window period," which normally lasts anywhere from three to six months after initial exposure. After the window period, these tests are highly accurate in detecting HIV.

Q: Could you tell me more about this window period? If a person has had unprotected sex, how soon can he be tested to be sure he hasn't contracted HIV?

A: The most difficult thing to grasp about the HIV test for many people is the concept of the window period. Most people infected with HIV begin producing detectable levels of antibodies by the third month, but some may take as long as six months. So the window period, in effect, runs from day 1 of infection to day 180. During this time, an antibody test *might not be* a valid diagnostic tool. *After* the window period—that is, after six months—the antibody test result can be viewed with confidence.

If a person is certain she has waited six months after the last act of unprotected sex, another test is unnecessary. If a person is unsure, though, getting retested would tell for certain whether the virus is present.

Regardless of your HIV status, you might want to get tested for other, more widespread STDs.

Q: I have heard about the over-the-counter HIV test kits. How do they work? Are they as reliable as a test in a doctor's office?

A: These kits allow a person to take a small blood sample from the fingertip, mail it to a designated laboratory for analysis and then get lab results by telephone, along with professional counseling and referrals if needed. The technology used to analyze samples is essentially the same as that used for standard in-clinic tests: analyzing the sample for antibodies to HIV. A positive test result with these kits is considered 99 percent accurate.

Some consumers have worried about the chance of samples getting mixed up at the lab, but this is even less likely with the home collection kits than with in-clinic tests. (One brand was taken off the market by its manufacturer, but this was due to poor sales rather than test performance.) So that the test can be anonymous, the kits use a unique personal identification number—one patient, one number—which guarantees that the number and the sample cannot be separated.

Critics have complained about the lack of face-to-face counseling with the home collection kits, but it seems likely that the fast-changing arena of rapid diagnostic tests will produce other "home tests" for STDs in the years to come.

Q: **What determines the difference between HIV disease and AIDS?**

A: A person who has HIV infection is diagnosed with AIDS based on testing for a specific type of cell produced by the immune system, the CD^4 T cell. A healthy adult will usually have a test score of 1,000 or more, but as HIV progresses, this number will drop. When it falls below 200, a person is diagnosed with AIDS. This diagnosis also can be made based on the presence of certain opportunistic infections.

Q: **How is HIV treated?**

A: When AIDS first appeared, the only approach was to treat symptoms alone because no drugs were available to combat the underlying viral infection. Over the past decade, however, therapies have been developed to fight both HIV infection and its associated infections and cancers.

The first group of drugs approved to treat HIV infection, called nucleoside reverse transcriptase (RT) inhibitors, interrupt an early stage of viral replication. Included in this class of drugs are AZT (zidovudine, brand name Retrovir), ddC (zalcitabine, brand name Hivid) and ddI. These drugs may slow the spread of HIV in the body and delay the onset of opportunistic infections.

Later, a second class of drugs called protease inhibitors was approved. These interrupt virus replication at a later step in its life cycle. They include ritonavir (Norvir), saquinivir (Invirase), indinavir (Crixivan) and nelfinavir (Viracept). Because HIV can become resistant to both classes of drugs, combination treatment using both is necessary to effectively suppress the virus.

The most recent additions to the list of HIV therapies are nonnucleoside reverse transcriptase inhibitors such as nevirapine (Viramune) and delavirdine (Rescriptor). These are sometimes used in combination with AZT.

Q: So can AIDS be effectively cured?

A: These drugs extend the life and improve the health of people with AIDS, but they do not cure AIDS or eliminate the underlying HIV infection. People taking these therapies can still transmit the disease.

Q: Is the HIV/AIDS epidemic over? Is it mainly now a problem among drug users?

A: The predicted expansion of the epidemic into the heterosexual population has occurred rather slowly and on a smaller scale than some researchers originally predicted. In 1998, rates of HIV infection *accelerated* faster among adolescents and heterosexual women than any other groups of people, but the largest *numbers* of infected individuals are found among injecting drug users who share needles and among gay men.

It would be comforting to think that the HIV epidemic will soon die out altogether, but the facts don't support this idea. For one thing, as our initial bout with AIDS has shown, we live in an interconnected world, and rates of HIV infection remain high in some segments of the U.S. population and in many parts of the globe, particularly in Africa and parts of Asia. Perhaps more important, in industrial countries, our major breakthroughs in treating AIDS may have the effect of lessening concern about preventing it. An increase in risky sex may regenerate the epidemic.

SAFER SEX

Q: What advice would you give to a person who is just becoming sexually active and wants to avoid getting an STD?

A: In truth, there is no simple one-size-fits-all strategy for avoiding STDs. The best approach is probably to start by understanding the factors that determine your risk of acquiring an STD and then to think about the precautions you might take to lower it.

As far as the first point, the basic principle is this: The more sexual partners you have, the more likely you are to acquire a sexually transmitted disease. Herpes is a good example. Among people who so far have had only one sexual partner, 10 percent are infected. Among those with five to nine partners, the number is 26 percent. Among those with 10 to 49 partners, it's 31 percent.

Making decisions about risk of STDs requires that you know something about your partner's history—how many people that person has had sex with, any past history of STDs and so on.

Q: So what can a person do—other than stay celibate?

A: The most effective all-around form of protection against STDs is the use of condoms for penetrative sexual acts such as vaginal or anal intercourse. They should also be used for **fellatio** (oral stimulation of the male genitalia). Condoms provide a barrier between the penis and the susceptible mucous membranes of the vagina, cervix, anus and mouth and stop the exchange of potentially infectious fluids such as semen, vaginal secretions, blood and stool.

This is true of the traditional male latex condom and also the newer polyurethane condoms, including the female condom that came onto the market in the mid-1990s. Lambskin condoms do offer some protection against STDs, but during the 1980s, research showed that microscopic pores in these devices were actually larger than some of the sexually transmitted viruses such as hepatitis B and HIV. For this reason, public health officials began to specify use of latex condoms in their efforts to stop the spread of HIV and other STDs. The newer polyurethane condoms haven't been studied as thoroughly as latex condoms, and they appear to have higher failure rates. This is discussed further in chapter 5.

Q: When are condoms effective and when aren't they?

A: Used properly and consistently, condoms can stop the spread of many infections, including chlamydia, gonorrhea, trichomoniasis, syphilis, hepatitis and HIV. Their effectiveness against the viral STDs herpes and HPV, however, is not completely known. The reason is that these two STDs can be spread readily from lesions that occur in places not covered or protected by a condom. For example, even if he were wearing a condom, a man with a herpes sore on the scrotum would put a female partner at risk because the close contact of intercourse might allow the virus to spread from scrotum to labia.

The phrase "properly and consistently" also bears on the effectiveness of condoms. Condoms, regardless of the material, can fail in a number of ways if misused. They can slip off if lubricated on the inside, for example, or if an erection subsides. And latex condoms can be damaged by use of oil-based lubricants such as hand creams, skin lotions and petroleum jelly. The female condom may take practice to insert correctly and can be dislodged in a number of ways. Proper use of the female condom is covered in chapter 5.

This is *not* to say that you have to be a rocket scientist to use condoms correctly. You do not. They are not only inexpensive and widely available but also easy to use. It's simply a good idea to familiarize yourself with the package insert of your brand to make sure your condom habits are correct.

Q: What are the most important guidelines on using condoms correctly?

A: Here are some tips:

- Store condoms in a cool, dark place. Heat and humidity are especially bad for latex.
- When opening a condom wrapper, be careful not to damage the condom itself with teeth, fingernails or jewelry.

- When putting on a condom, hold the tip—the part where semen will be deposited—between the thumb and forefinger and squeeze out any air bubbles that may be present, including any air in a reservoir-style tip.
- Do not use oil-based lubricants such as household skin lotions because they can damage latex condoms. Water-based lubricants such as K-Y Jelly and Astroglide are safe.
- Unroll the condom over the entire shaft of the penis.
- After penetrative intercourse, remove the penis while it's still erect; otherwise, the condom may slip off prematurely.

Q: What about spermicides?

A: Spermicides, as the term implies, were developed as a contraceptive—to kill sperm. It was later discovered in laboratory experiments that they also kill some of the microbes associated with STDs, and some research has shown that they can help prevent the transmission of chlamydia and gonorrhea. Against this backdrop, some have advocated the use of spermicides as a form of STD prevention for those who will not or cannot use condoms. This is still a controversial recommendation, however, because if used often, spermicides can cause irritation in the vagina. In addition, there are questions about the proper dose needed to neutralize or kill STDs, which may be different from the dose that works to kill sperm.

Q: Is oral sex safer—that is, less likely to spread STDs—than other kinds of penetrative sex?

A: In a general sense, yes. Most STDs have the potential to be spread through oral sex, most commonly resulting in sore throat and other oral symptoms. But it's also true, as a rule, that sexually transmitted infections in the mouth and throat are much less likely to develop than genital infections, which suggests a lower risk from oral sex. This may be because the oral cavity is a less hospitable environment for sexually transmitted microbes than the genital tract, though this remains a matter of speculation.

Oral sex, however, does account for substantial numbers of sexually transmitted diseases, including gonorrhea and herpes.

It is also still considered a risk for HIV, specifically because of the potential for cuts or abrasions in the gums that might give HIV an open door into the bloodstream.

In sum, the risk from oral sex is lower than having penetrative vaginal or anal intercourse, but it isn't zero. For this reason, people practicing oral sex with a partner who might carry an STD are advised to use condoms for fellatio or barriers such as dental dams and plastic wrap for cunnilingus.

Q: What's a dental dam?

A: Originally developed for use in oral surgery, dental dams are square pieces of thin latex that can also be used to prevent the exchange of body fluids during oral sex. A dam must be held in position over the vulva or anus during oral stimulation, always keeping the same side of the dam against the body.

Dental dams can be purchased through various sex boutiques and catalogs. Some authorities recommend plastic wrap as an alternative to dental dams because it's easier to get and can be used in larger sizes.

Q: What is outercourse—and is it safe?

A: Outercourse is a term coined in the 1980s as part of the effort to prevent the spread of HIV by encouraging safer sex. It refers generally to practices that can give sexual pleasure without creating the risks implicit in vaginal, oral or anal sex. Examples include sensual massage, fantasy, self-masturbation, pleasuring a partner with the hands and other forms of sex play. Safety is a relative issue. Although much safer than penetrative sex, some forms of outercourse do carry the risk of skin-to-skin transmission for herpes or genital HPV. The following chart, adapted from a brochure titled "As Safe As You Wanna Be," from the AIDS Prevention Project in Seattle, Washington, ranks two dozen sexual acts according to levels of risk for acquiring HIV. Its message is quite appropriate: Different activities will have different levels of acceptable risk. It falls to each individual to decide where to draw the line.

Sexual Activities and Their HIV Risk

NO RISK:
Hugging; massage; clothed body rubbing; masturbation; fantasy; dry kissing; unshared sex toys; use of a hot tub, bath or sauna

VERY LOW RISK:
Intercourse between the thighs; oral sex on a man without taking the head of the penis into the mouth; masturbating a partner while using latex gloves or while having no cuts or broken skin; giving or receiving oral sex with a latex condom or barrier; deep kissing; sharing sex toys and using disinfection, cleaning or new condoms

LOW RISK:
Insertive vaginal or anal intercourse (if you're a man, your penis in someone's vagina or rectum) with a condom; receiving oral sex without a latex barrier

MEDIUM RISK:
Sharing sex toys without using disinfection, cleaning or new condoms; inserting your finger or hand with cuts into a vagina or anus; receptive anal or vaginal intercourse (someone's penis in your rectum or, if you're a woman, your vagina) with a condom; giving oral sex without a latex barrier; breast milk in the mouth

HIGH RISK:
Insertive vaginal or anal intercourse without a condom

HIGHEST RISK:
Receptive vaginal or anal intercourse without a condom

Source: The AIDS Prevention Project, Seattle-King County Department of Public Health, April 1995.

Q: **What if a person already has an STD? How can the person's partner get protection?**

A: Again, there's no universal measure to stop all STDs. With infections that can be cured with medication, the person would ideally refrain from having sex until the infection is cleared. With chronic infections such as genital herpes or genital HPV, it's wise to avoid contact with lesions, but—as we stressed earlier—these infections can be transmitted even when no obvious lesions are present. So if you have herpes or HPV, you should talk the issues through with your partner and decide which precautions, if any, you need to take.

Q: **What about a woman who has had only a couple of sexual partners and whose annual gynecological exams have always been normal? Should she still be concerned about having a sexually transmitted disease?**

A: Although her partners' sexual histories are a significant factor, too, the good news is that, as far as statistics are concerned, a women with only a couple of partners stands a lower chance of contracting an STD than someone who has a larger number of partners. The fact that her annual Pap smears and gynecological exams have been normal and that she reports no troubling symptoms raise the likelihood that she is free of STDs.

On the other hand, as we have stressed, a number of very widespread STDs tend to be asymptomatic. And annual gynecological exams do not routinely include screening for STDs. Therefore, one can't be entirely sure about being free of STDs based simply on routine care. Chlamydia, as an example, is both extremely common and frequently silent. And as we said earlier, it can also affect a woman's ability to have children, which is why it's a good idea for all sexually active women to be screened for chlamydia.

Screening can also be done for other STDs in their asymptomatic phases, including herpes. It's a good idea to talk with your health care provider about your situation and which, if any, tests might be needed.

STDs During Pregnancy

Several STDs can be spread to babies either in the womb or at birth, including herpes, genital warts, chlamydia, gonorrhea, HIV and syphilis. Some STDs can be transmitted to infants after birth through direct skin contact with lesions—for example, through a kiss from an adult who has a cold sore. In order to protect babies from possible gonorrhea infection, it is standard practice in delivery rooms to administer eye drops of silver nitrate or erythromycin oinment to all newborns. The later therapy also works to prevent chlamydia in newborns.

If you are pregnant, be sure that your baby doesn't become infected. Report any STD to your health care provider—and be sure it's treated. In many cases, testing for STDs such as chlamydia, gonorrhea and syphilis is a standard part of prenatal care, and HIV testing should be offered as well. But if you have a history of any STD, it's a good idea to inquire about it.

Herpes testing is usually not a part of routine prenatal care, so if you are a woman who has herpes or whose partner has this infection, it's advisable to discuss with your ob-gyn or nurse-midwife what precautions could be taken to avert the risk of infecting the child.

The second major caveat is to avoid becoming infected with an STD during pregnancy. All of the STDs we have listed here, including common infections such as herpes, can cause serious illness and sometimes permanent damage in newborns. With herpes in particular, it is the mothers with *newly acquired* infections who are most likely to infect their infants. Any woman who has a partner with genital herpes but who is not infected herself should take precautions to avoid acquiring herpes during pregnancy. This will include avoiding contact with any herpes lesions, using condoms for all acts of intercourse and possibly abstaining from sexual intercourse during the third trimester.

Q: How can I tell if my prospective sexual partner has an STD?

A: You can't always tell, but you can always ask. We live in an age when STDs are a big issue. If you're contemplating a sexual relationship with a new partner, ideally you should discuss past sexual experiences and sexually transmitted diseases—first. For most people, the concern driving this discussion *and* driving the need for condom use or other safer-sex approaches has been the fear of AIDS. But as long as you're talking about AIDS, you might as well talk about the other STDs that are more common than AIDS.

Of course, talking about it carries no guarantees. There are those who will lie and those who quite honestly don't know that they have an STD. Most people who have genital herpes, for example, never experience obvious symptoms—likewise with chlamydia.

If you are sexually involved with someone, don't turn a blind eye to any type of rash, sore or ulcer in the genital area. Likewise, cold sores or fever blisters on or around the lips pose a risk of transmitting herpes through oral sex.

If you are frequently having sex with people you don't really know and with whom you have not had an in-depth discussion about safer sex, the proper use of condoms or other barriers (such as dental dams) is in order. Also remember that alcohol and recreational drug use—while they may reduce inhibition—can interfere with the ability to make smart choices about safer sex.

Q: How do I tell my partner I have an STD?

A: Telling a prospective partner you have an STD can be difficult for those who have a persistent viral infection such as herpes, genital HPV or hepatitis. Bringing up your personal history with one of these infections is probably easiest in the context of a more inclusive safer-sex conversation. Before you become involved with anyone sexually, you deserve to know something of that person's sexual history. You have news to share, and perhaps your potential partner does, too.

Choose a quiet, private place with a relaxed, nonsexual atmosphere and try to ensure that you have ample time for discussion. It's normal to feel apprehensive about explaining your condition, and it's normal for your partner to feel apprehensive about the possibility of contracting an infection. Remember that most people have a poor understanding of what STDs are, how common they are, how they're transmitted and how they're treated.

Be prepared to answer questions, and don't expect your partner to come to terms with the issue on the spot. Give your partner time to take it all in.

4 OTHER REPRODUCTIVE AND URINARY TRACT DISORDERS

Q: Are there any other reproductive or urinary tract disorders that the average woman or man should know about?

A: There are several. Women need to be aware of bacterial vaginosis, yeast infection (officially called vulvovaginal candidiasis, or VVC) and urinary tract infection. Men should be familiar with **prostatitis** and **prostate cancer** (conditions affecting the prostate gland), **Peyronie's disease** (a condition of the penis), epididymitis (inflammation of tubular structures connected to the testes), **orchitis** (inflammation of the testes), **testicular cancer, testicular torsion** and **hydrocele**.

PROBLEMS AND CONCERNS FOR WOMEN

Bacterial Vaginosis

Q: What's the difference between vaginitis and bacterial vaginosis? I've seen both terms used to describe vaginal infection.

A: Strictly speaking, the suffix *itis* is used to indicate inflammation (pain, redness and swelling). The suffix *osis* is used to describe a more generalized state of disease or infection and does not imply inflammation. Vaginitis, then, is an inflammation of vaginal tissues caused by various microbes; as we explain in chapter 3, these include the sexually transmitted microbe trichomonas. Bacterial vaginosis (BV) is an abnormal and excessive colonization of the vagina by various kinds of *undesirable bacteria*. It is not usually accompanied by pain, redness or swelling of vaginal tissues. The main point is that with vaginitis, bacteria cause inflammation. With BV, undesirable bacteria are present, but instead of inflammation, they may cause abnormal odor or excessive discharge.

Q: I'm a little confused by that phrase "undesirable bacteria." Aren't all bacteria undesirable in the vagina, and shouldn't a woman try to keep her vagina as free of bacteria as possible?

A: No! That's the last thing a woman should do. Just like the healthy mouth or the healthy gut, the healthy vagina always contains a large variety of different types of bacteria. Having the right kinds of bacteria present in the right proportions is not only normal but also essential for good vaginal health.

The predominant species of bacteria found in the healthy vagina are of the genus *Lactobacillus*—bacteria that produce lactic acid as one of their by-products. The predominance of lactobacilli—at least some types of them—is thought to help prevent infection by other bacteria.

It may surprise you to learn that from a bacterial standpoint a healthy vagina is much cleaner than the human mouth. This means that douching is never necessary unless prescribed by a doctor. Over-the-counter (OTC) douches sold in drugstores and grocery stores do *nothing* to promote vaginal health. In fact, these products actually contribute to the overgrowth of undesirable bacteria and may increase the risk of pelvic inflammatory disease and other problems.

Q: If the vagina is normally so full of bacteria, how is that situation any different from BV?

A: The critical difference is in the kinds of bacteria present. When we talk about bacteria in the vagina (or the gut or the mouth), we often use the expression "normal **flora**." This refers to the complex mix of microorganisms that are normally found at these sites in more-or-less stable ratios. As noted earlier, lactobacilli are the most common bacteria in the healthy vagina. What we see in BV is a decline in the number of lactobacilli and an overgrowth of various "bad" bacteria, such as *Gardnerella vaginalis, Mycoplasma hominis* and various species of anaerobic bacteria (bacteria that live and grow in the absence of oxygen). Streptococci also have been associated with BV. All of these bacterial species may be found in small numbers in the healthy vagina. In BV, they are present in abnormally large numbers, to the detriment of the lactobacilli.

Another issue is the particular species of lactobacilli present in the vagina. The vaginal lactobacilli found in women *without BV* are usually of the species that produce hydrogen peroxide (H_2O_2) as a by-product. This H_2O_2 is believed to help inhibit the growth of the "bad" bacteria listed above. Women with BV tend to have vaginal lactobacilli that do not produce H_2O_2.

Q: What causes the vaginal flora to go out of balance?

A: Exactly why this happens is not known. The healthy vagina has been compared with a complex ecosystem supporting a number of life forms in a state of balance. Imagine, just for example, a pristine woodland pond. In and around this pond, numerous plants and animals coexist. Now imagine that somehow a new species of aquatic algae is introduced into the pond—an algae with no natural enemies. Over time, this new algae grows and grows, filling the pond and covering its surface. Eventually, the other aquatic plants are crowded out; they cannot compete for sunlight or oxygen. The fish suffocate. The plant-eating animals die off or leave, as do the animals that depend on the plant-eating animals as a source of food. Where once we had a complex and balanced little ecosystem, we now have a stagnant, algae-choked pond. Current thinking on the causes of BV suggests that a roughly similar phenomenon occurs when a particular collection of "bad" bacteria is *introduced* into the vagina; the newcomers grow out of control, spoil the formerly well-balanced vaginal environment and make it impossible for other, beneficial bacteria to survive. What is less clear, however, is what causes the bacteria that are normally present in the vagina in small quantities to suddenly grow out of control.

Q: Are there any known risk factors for developing BV?

A: One factor identified as predisposing women to the development of BV is the use of an **intrauterine device (IUD)** for contraception. BV is also associated with some of the same risk factors as sexually transmitted diseases—specifically, multiple sex partners and recent intercourse with a new partner.

Q: Is BV a sexually transmitted disease?

A: Some cases are sexually transmitted. In one study, women seeking treatment at an STD clinic were found to be about twice as likely to have BV as women with similar symptoms who sought treatment at a family practice clinic. The principal microbe associated with BV, *Gardnerella vaginalis,* is far more likely to be found in the vaginas of sexually active women than in sexually inexperienced women. Also, *G. vaginalis* has been found in the urethras of 79 to 86 percent of the male sex partners of women with BV. (It's not clear in such cases which partner is the source of the infection.) These men's urethras may also be colonized with the other bacteria associated with BV.

Q: How common is BV?

A: Overall, it has been estimated that 25 percent of women seen at ob-gyn clinics around the country have BV; it is the most common cause of vaginal symptoms (of any kind) in women of childbearing age.

Q: How would a woman know if she had BV?

A: She might not be able to tell—about 50 percent of women with BV have no obvious signs or symptoms. The classic signs of BV are a white or light gray vaginal discharge and a distinctly fishlike vaginal odor. At least one of these signs is present in about half of all cases. The discharge, usually found in amounts only slightly greater than the normal volume of vaginal discharge, has a uniform consistency and isn't particularly thick. About a third of women with BV describe their vaginal discharge as yellow in color. Vaginal malodor (the fishy smell) may be especially pronounced immediately after intercourse.

Q: How is BV diagnosed?

A: Presence of the characteristic discharge will raise a health care provider's index of suspicion, but there are other conditions that also cause vaginal discharge, including trichomoniasis and yeast infection. Regarding vaginal malodor, there is a clinical test that entails mixing a drop of vaginal fluid with a drop of potassium hydroxide solution to more fully release the compounds responsible for the fishy smell. However, as a diagnostic technique, this so-called whiff test is considerably less reliable than microscopic examination. And again, only about 50 percent of women with BV have the discharge or the fishy vaginal odor.

Almost all women with BV have a vaginal pH greater than 4.5. (The normal range is 4.0 to 4.5.) In addition, the microscopic evaluation of vaginal fluid from a woman with BV will usually reveal what are called "clue cells"—vaginal cells whose outer edges are encrusted with bacteria such as *G. vaginalis*. Clue cells are present in up to 81 percent of cases.

A composite diagnosis of BV should be based on the presence of three of these four features: characteristic discharge; "fishy" smell from vaginal fluid mixed with potassium hydroxide solution; vaginal pH greater than 4.5; and clue cells.

Q: How is BV treated?

A: Oral antibiotics such as metronidazole (brand names include Flagyl, Metizol and Prostat) and clindamycin (Cleocin) have been the standard treatments for many years. Both are now available by prescription as intravaginal creams. Used for seven days, these creams are just as effective as oral therapy and produce fewer side effects. Some researchers have proposed a one-dose treatment consisting of 2 grams of oral metronidazole, but this has a slightly lower cure rate than the weeklong regimens.

Q: How effective is antibacterial therapy for BV?

A: Unfortunately, recurrences are common. For example, up to 80 percent of women with BV who are successfully treated with metronidazole experience a recurrence of the infection within nine months. We don't know why. Possible explanations include the following:

- Reinfection by a male sex partner who carries the bacteria responsible for BV

- Persistence of "bad" bacteria that were inhibited but not killed by antibiotic therapy
- Failure to reestablish the normal mix of vaginal flora, especially lactobacilli, after therapy
- Persistence of an as-yet unidentified factor, such as allergy or improper nutrition, that makes the woman susceptible to reinfection

Q: Are OTC products that contain lactobacillus effective in the treatment of BV?

A: Probably not. Many women believe that drinking acidophilus milk, eating yogurt or taking various lactobacillus-containing capsules and powders sold in health food stores will restore the proper balance of lactobacilli to the vagina. There is no good research to indicate that this is true. Some women actually apply yogurt directly into the vagina, but this practice cannot be recommended. The reason is that bacteria tend to be closely adapted to their particular ecological niche. Commercial strains of dairy lactobacilli have been shown to adhere poorly to the vaginal walls and are unlikely to successfully colonize the vagina. It's also important to note that more than 50 percent of the lactobacillus preparations available in the United States have been shown to be contaminated with other bacteria.

Q: If BV goes untreated, what are the possible consequences?

A: Aside from the anxiety or self-consciousness that may accompany vaginal discharge or odor, BV is also linked with a number of obstetric and gynecologic complications. Some have to do with pregnancy outcome—for example, increased risk of preterm labor and low birthweight babies. BV also has been implicated in other reproductive tract problems such as pelvic inflammatory disease and ectopic pregnancy, both of which are discussed in chapter 3. Ectopic pregnancy occurs when the pregnancy develops outside the uterus, usually in the fallopian tube. It is always a serious condition and can be fatal in some cases.

Lastly, BV has been associated with increased risk of gonorrhea and of acquiring the human immunodeficiency virus (HIV).

Q: Should every woman with BV be treated?

A: Although a number of complications have been linked with BV, the degree of risk has not been firmly established, and there is no flat recommendation that all women with BV be treated. Many cases have gone untreated because they caused no discharge and no odor. Some women are aware of the discharge and odor but accept it as normal because they have been living with the problem for years and didn't realize the cause. At the very least, a woman with BV should be advised of the possible complications and offered the option of antibacterial therapy.

Some clinicians advocate treating all pregnant women who have BV, but others caution about possible risk to the fetus from antibiotic toxicity. The Centers for Disease Control and Prevention recommends that all women who have previously given birth to a premature baby be screened for BV and treated with oral metronidazole or oral clindamycin if the diagnosis is positive.

Q: Should male sex partners of women with BV be treated?

A: The jury is still out on this question. Despite the fact that up to 86 percent of the male sex partners of women with BV have *G. vaginalis* in their urethras, no study to date has convincingly shown that treating these partners reduces the rate of recurrent infection in women. However, if a woman experiences several recurrences of BV, treating her male partner to eliminate *G. vaginalis* and other bacteria from his urethra may be helpful.

Q: Can BV be prevented?

A: Given the association of BV with heterosexual intercourse, two obvious lines of defense are abstinence and the use of condoms. Barring these precautions, however, there is little to recommend in the way of prevention. We don't really know how the intravaginal environment becomes unbalanced, so we don't know how to prevent it.

Women would do well to keep the following facts in mind. It has been reported that 80 percent of women do not know the signs of BV. Many women mistake BV for a yeast infection and self-medicate inappropriately. Seventy percent of women treat vaginal infections with OTC medications before seeking professional help, but as noted earlier, OTC medications are effectively useless against BV. Nearly half the women surveyed by the American Social Health Association said that their health care providers *did not* screen for vaginal infections during routine exams, and one-third reported that they were not asked about unusual vaginal discharge or odor. Women who experience one or both of these classic symptoms of BV (or who have experienced them in the past) should raise the issue of BV with their practitioners.

Yeast Infection (Vulvovaginal Candidiasis)

Q: What's the difference between bacterial vaginosis and a yeast infection?

A: The biggest difference is the cause. Bacterial vaginosis, as the name implies, is a bacterial infection. A yeast infection—vulvovaginal candidiasis (VVC)—is fungal. Yeasts are single-cell fungi. Between 85 and 90 percent of the yeasts found in the vagina are of one species, *Candida albicans,* and this causes almost all cases of VVC. Other candida species can also cause yeast infections, including *Candida glabatra* and another yeast called *Torulopsis.*

We use the term "vulvovaginal" to specify the site because candida can also infect the mouth and throat. The resulting oral candidiasis is sometimes called **thrush** and most commonly affects infants and people with compromised immune systems (cancer patients, transplant patients and AIDS patients, for example).

It is possible for a woman to have bacterial vaginosis and VVC at the same time.

Q: Where does the yeast come from, and is there any way to keep it out of the vagina?

A: Candida appears to occur naturally among the normal flora of the gut, and given the vagina's proximity to the anus, the source of candida colonizing the vagina is thought to be that region. The presence of candida is not the same as VVC;

it has been estimated that about 20 percent of women with no evidence of VVC nonetheless have candida in their vaginas.

Q: How widespread a problem is VVC?

A: In the United States, VVC is the second most common form of vaginal infection after bacterial vaginosis. It has been estimated that 75 percent of all women will experience at least one episode of symptomatic VVC in their lifetimes. In tropical and subtropical countries with warm climates, it is often the number-one form of vaginal infection. Most experts agree that VVC is on the rise in this country, and they attribute the increase mainly to the widespread use of antibiotics.

Q: What is the connection between VVC and the use of antibiotics?

A: The oral and topical antibiotics used to treat bacterial vaginal infection are highly effective at eliminating bacteria. But as we explained earlier in the section of this chapter dealing with bacterial vaginosis, vaginal health depends on the balanced presence of a number of bacterial species, especially lactobacilli. It's not unusual to find relatively small numbers of candida in the healthy vagina, but they are inhibited and controlled by the normal vaginal bacteria. Antibiotics reduce or eliminate some of the normal vaginal bacteria, upsetting the balance of microbes we described earlier. Sometimes an overgrowth of candida results.

Q: In addition to the use of vaginal antibiotics, are there any other factors that predispose a woman to develop VVC?

A: Several risk factors for VVC have been identified. First, it has been linked to high estrogen levels: Girls who have not started menstruating and women who have completed menopause rarely get VVC. On the other hand, pregnant women (who have very high estrogen levels) and women taking high-estrogen birth control pills are more likely to develop VVC. Candida infection is also more common in women with uncontrolled diabetes and in those with impaired immune systems.

The wearing of tight, poorly ventilated clothing and underpants made from nylon or some other fabric that doesn't "breathe" predisposes a woman to the development of VVC by increasing heat and moisture in the crotch area.

Lastly, there is some evidence that commercial douches, perfumed toilet paper, chlorinated swimming-pool water, so-called feminine hygiene sprays and spermicides contribute to the development of VVC. The chemicals in these products may cause allergic reactions in the vaginal tissue or cause a decrease in lactobacilli that triggers an overgrowth of candida.

Q: What are the symptoms of VVC?

A: Some women will have no symptoms. When symptoms are present, the most common is itching of the external vaginal tissues, known as **vulvar pruritis**. Vaginal discharge is also fairly common; it is usually described as "cottage cheeselike" but may vary in consistency from watery to thick. Unlike bacterial vaginosis, VVC is often accompanied by inflammation. Vulvar burning, vaginal soreness and irritation, pain during intercourse (dyspareunia) and pain during urination (**dysuria**) are common, as are redness and swelling of the labia and other vulvar tissues. Unlike BV, VVC is not associated with malodor; if present at all, odor is usually mild and inoffensive. The symptoms of VVC tend to worsen in the week immediately preceding a menstrual period and lessen with the onset of menstrual flow.

Male sex partners of women with VVC may experience penile rash, redness and itching a few minutes to a few hours after vaginal intercourse without a condom. These effects usually disappear after the male partner bathes or showers. A woman whose partner experiences these symptoms should consider the possibility that she has VVC.

Q: Can't men get yeast infections also?

A: Yes. It is more common among **uncircumcised** men, as infection finds an ideal environment under the foreskin. Another common site of yeast infection in men—**circumcised** or uncircumcised—is in the groin, at the junction of the scrotum and upper thighs.

Q: Is VVC transmitted sexually? Should male sex partners of women with recurrent VVC be treated?

A: Candida is found in 20 percent of the male sex partners of women with recurrent VVC, a rate four times higher than that seen in the male population at large. While some degree of sexual transmission seems likely, its role remains unclear. As a result, it is not standard practice to treat the male partners of women with recurrent VVC.

Q: How is VVC diagnosed?

A: A diagnosis of VVC requires correlation among clinical signs and symptoms, microscopic findings and vaginal culture. The simplest and most reliable diagnostic technique is microscopic examination of vaginal fluid, which also helps rule out other vaginal infections such as bacterial vaginosis and trichomoniasis. However, the failure to find candida under microscopic examination does not rule out VVC. A vaginal culture should be performed if the microscopic evaluation is negative. Many women are misdiagnosed with VVC on the basis of symptoms or vaginal culture alone. The symptoms of VVC can mimic those of other vaginal infections and conditions, and culture methods *alone* are unreliable because so many women carry *Candida* as part of their normal vaginal flora.

A rapid, in-office test for VVC has been developed by the National Institute of Allergy and Infectious Disease and should be available soon.

Q: Should all women with VVC be treated, and if so, how?

A: Physicians usually recommend against treating women with VVC that causes no symptoms. When treatment is needed, however, roughly a dozen different antifungals are available, including nystatin (Mycostatin, Nilstat), miconazole (Monistat), clotrimazole (Lotrimin, Mycelex), tioconazole (Vagistat-1) and butoconazole (Femstat). These creams, tablets and suppositories are administered intravaginally for three to seven days. A single oral dose of fluconazole (Diflucan) is also effective and preferred by some women for its convenience.

In general, women who are subject to recurrent VVC should be treated with a longer course of therapy.

Several of the antifungals listed above are available in non-prescription versions; however, a cautionary note is needed here. VVC is hard to diagnose. At one clinic specializing in VVC, more than 80 percent of the women referred, *by their doctors,* for treatment of chronic or recurrent VVC were found not to have VVC at all, but vaginitis due to some other cause. Given the difficulty of diagnosing VVC, even for the trained physician, self-diagnosis and self-treatment of what seems like VVC may simply the delay the treatment of another, more serious vaginal infection. If you have a problem with chronic or recurring VVC and your doctor approves the use of an OTC antifungal, that's fine. They *are* effective. In other circumstances, it's not advisable to self-diagnose and self-medicate VVC or any vaginal infection.

Q: How effective are the available treatments for VVC?

A: Studies suggest a 70 to 80 percent cure rate with nystatin. The topical imidazoles (miconazole, clotrimazole and so on) are 80 to 90 percent effective when administered for five to seven days.

It has been found that roughly one out of four women will never develop VVC. Of those women who experience at least one episode, 40 to 50 percent will have at least one recurrence, and some will have repeated, recurrent and often chronic VVC. Why VVC recurs so easily among these women is still the subject of medical research.

Q: What can be done for women with recurrent VVC?

A: Recurrent VVC—defined as four or more episodes of clinically confirmed VVC in a 12-month period—can be frustrating to treat, but almost all cases of chronic VVC can be controlled, if not absolutely cured. The first steps involve the removal of any predisposing factors, including the following:

- Uncontrolled diabetes must be brought under control.
- Corticosteroids and other immunosuppressive agents should be discontinued if possible.

- Therapeutic estrogen should be stopped if possible.
- High-estrogen birth control pills should be discontinued (low-estrogen pills pose no apparent problems).
- Tight-fitting clothes should be avoided, and only cotton underpants should be worn.
- Douching, which is of no value anyway, should be discontinued.
- Use of a spermicidal birth control method should be stopped if possible.

Many women with chronic VVC self-medicate, treating each recurrent episode individually with a topical medication. A correctly diagnosed case of chronic VVC may instead require ongoing preventive therapy with an oral antifungal. It should be noted, though, that long-term antifungal therapy, even with the relatively safe agents available for VVC, may pose risks such as hepatitis.

Also, women prone to VVC who are undergoing antibacterial therapy for another infection should probably receive simultaneous therapy with a topical antifungal.

Q: Are there any women who should not be treated for VVC?

A: Pregnant women are among those who shouldn't be treated for VVC. Pregnant women are more susceptible to VVC than women who are not pregnant, and treatment has to be decided on a case-by-case basis. Physicians may be especially wary of exposing the fetus to antifungals in the first trimester of pregnancy because of the risk of toxicity. Most of the conventional topical antifungals are effective for pregnant women, but their infections are likely to require longer courses of therapy and are more likely to recur.

Q: What are the consequences of untreated VVC?

A: No serious long-term medical consequences have been identified, but the stress and anxiety of recurrent episodes of symptomatic VVC must be taken into account, especially the potential impact of painful sexual intercourse on intimate relationships.

Urinary Tract Infections

Q: What is a urinary tract infection?

A: The urinary tract includes all the organs and tissues involved in the manufacture, storage and elimination of urine—including the **kidneys**, the bladder and the urethra. A urinary tract infection (UTI) can involve any part or parts of this system; in this discussion, however, we use UTI to refer only to **urethritis** and **cystitis**—infections of the urethra and the bladder, respectively. We also distinguish between acute (sudden onset) and recurrent UTI because causes and treatments of each may vary.

One further distinction—the information in this section applies to *uncomplicated UTIs*—for example, those occurring in the absence of diabetes, a suppressed immune system, kidney disease, bladder obstruction or anatomic or functional abnormalities of the urinary tract.

Q: What are the symptoms of UTI?

A: Many cases produce no obvious symptoms, but the classic signs and symptoms include the following:

- Painful urination
- Feeling a strong need to urinate
- Needing to urinate often but only in small quantities
- Internal pain directly above the pubic region

Clinical evaluation of a urine specimen may reveal the presence of pus **(pyuria)**, blood **(hematuria)** and abnormally high numbers of "bad" bacteria **(bacteriuria)**.

Q: How common are UTIs?

A: UTIs affect both sexes but are much more common in women, accounting for more than 5 million doctors' office visits each year. UTIs are seen in only 1 to 3 percent of young girls. However, the incidence rises sharply among sexually active adolescents and is highest among young women 20 to 25 years of age.

Q: What causes UTIs?

A: While various microbes can infect the urethra and bladder, an estimated 80 percent of acute bacterial UTIs are caused by *Escherichia coli,* which is among the normal bacteria found in the gastrointestinal tract. The second most common cause of bacterial UTI is *Staphylococcus saprophyticus.* In either case, infection is frequently believed to spread from the anus to the nearby openings of the vagina and urethra. In almost all cases of bladder infection, bacteria gain entrance to the bladder via the urethra.

Q: Are UTIs sexually transmitted?

A: Urethritis is a fairly common feature of several STDs, including chlamydia, gonorrhea and genital herpes. In women, however, bacterial UTIs are generally not regarded as STDs.

This is not to say bacterial UTIs aren't related to sexual activity. Sexually active women are more prone to UTIs than women without sexual experience. This link has long been recognized, as evidenced in the terms "honeymoon cystitis" and "honeymoon bladder," used colloquially to describe an acute UTI that appears after the initiation of sexual activity. Bacteria from the area around the anus that are already present on vaginal surfaces are thought to be introduced into the bladder through the urethra by the massaging motion of vaginal intercourse. In fact, one thing sexually active women can do to reduce their risk of UTI is urinate immediately after intercourse to help flush these bacteria out of the urinary tract.

Q: Are there other factors that contribute to a woman's risk of UTI?

A: Regular use of a diaphragm and spermicide appears to increase a woman's risk of UTI by altering the balance of bacteria normally found in the entrance of the vagina, which in turn can lead to the overgrowth of the proverbial "bad" bacteria. In addition, a recent study has shown that the use of condoms coated with spermicide increases a woman's risk of UTI caused by *S. saprophyticus.* There is also evidence that condom use in general may—for unexplained reasons—elevate the risk of UTI. Although the relationship of condoms to UTIs is under study, it appears best to use lubricated condoms without spermicide if UTIs are a concern.

Q: How are UTIs diagnosed?

A: If classic signs and symptoms are present, with no complicating factors, microscopic evaluation of a urine specimen is often sufficient for diagnosis. If the diagnosis is positive, antibacterial therapy can be started. Culturing a urine specimen to determine which bacteria are present and then testing the bacteria to determine if they are susceptible to particular antibiotics may be necessary in some cases.

Q: How are UTIs treated?

A: Treatment of simple, uncomplicated UTIs is fairly straightforward. A short course of low-dose antibiotics is usually effective. Since more than 80 percent of acute uncomplicated bacterial cystitis is due to *E. coli,* a health care provider will probably prescribe one of several antibiotics known to be effective against *E. coli.* Single-dose regimens are often sufficient and offer the added value of convenience, lower cost and reduced potential for side effects. However, single-dose regimens are not as effective as three- to seven-day regimens in preventing recurrence, perhaps because they are not as efficient in clearing *E. coli* that have colonized the vagina.

Q: What about men and urinary tract infections?

A: Male urethritis is most often seen in connection with the STDs chlamydia and gonorrhea, as discussed in chapter 3. Symptoms of difficult urination and urethral discharge are also common among men with acute genital herpes infection. With the exception of UTIs associated with STDs, UTIs are rare in men younger than 50 years of age. In elderly men, however, bacteriuria—the finding of high concentrations of bacteria in the urine—is quite common. Let's now talk more about some of the problems that can affect men.

PROBLEMS AND CONCERNS FOR MEN

Prostatitis

Q: What about prostate infection? Isn't the prostate gland part of the male urinary tract?

A: In a way, yes, though it isn't involved directly in the manufacture, storage or elimination of urine. As we explained in chapter 2, the prostate gland is located immediately under the bladder. It completely surrounds the urethra and is connected to it by ducts, through which it pumps prostatic fluid (a milky, alkaline component of semen) during orgasm and ejaculation. When the prostate becomes inflamed, we call the condition prostatitis.

Q: What causes prostatitis?

A: That depends on what kind of prostatitis we're talking about. The medical literature recognizes three main types: acute bacterial prostatitis, chronic bacterial prostatitis and nonbacterial prostatitis. Nonbacterial prostatitis is further subdivided into prostatodynia ("painful prostate") and congestive prostatitis. Since congestive prostatitis is the most common form, let's take a look at it first.

Congestive prostatitis occurs when too much prostatic fluid builds up in the prostate. Most experts think this buildup is linked to sexual activity or, in some cases, to a lack of sexual activity. Congestive prostatitis has been called "the disease of popes and priests," the implication being that men who do not ejaculate on a regular basis are more likely to experience an excessive buildup of prostatic fluid. Ironically, though, the condition also sometimes afflicts men who have sex regularly and ejaculate frequently. These men have prostates that are conditioned to produce a larger amount of prostatic fluid than men who are celibate or have sex infrequently. Problems may occur, however, if these men stop having sex regularly and stop ejaculating. This is because the prostate goes on producing prostatic fluid at the same rate as before, and the fluid may accumulate.

Q: What are the symptoms of congestive prostatitis?

A: A man with congestive prostatitis often finds that the opening of his penis is stuck together in the morning when he wakes up. When he unsticks it, a couple of drops of clear fluid can be seen. By day's end, a man may find a yellow-to-brown stain about an inch in diameter on the front of his underpants. Some men complain of an itching sensation deep inside the penis. Discomfort during urination is common. Physical examination may reveal that the prostate is swollen, and since the urethra passes right through the middle of the prostate, this swelling may hinder the passage of urine.

Q: How does prostatodynia differ from congestive prostatitis, and what causes it?

A: Prostatodynia is diagnosed when the signs and symptoms of congestive prostatitis are present without bacteriuria or clinical evidence of inflammation. Prostatodynia may also cause pain or discomfort in the rectum, in the **perineum** (the area between the anus and the scrotum) or internally and just above the pubic hair. We don't know for sure what causes prostatodynia. It may be stress-related. In some cases, prostatodynia is associated with an overly tense **urinary sphincter** (one of the muscles that controls the flow of urine).

Q: How are congestive prostatitis and prostatodynia treated?

A: If your health care provider suspects congestive rather than bacterial prostatitis, she may massage your prostate in the course of the examination to help expel the built-up prostatic fluid. It is also recommended that you find the means to ejaculate, either by intercourse or by masturbation, to reduce the pressure from excess fluid.

Since stress appears to be a possible cause of prostatodynia, tranquilizers, psychotherapy and other stress-reducing measures may be useful. You may also be offered muscle relaxants to counter excess tone in the urinary sphincter muscle.

Q: What about acute and chronic bacterial prostatitis? Are the signs and symptoms the same as for congestive prostatitis?

A: With acute bacterial prostatitis, in addition to the symptoms of congestive prostatitis, you may also have chills, fever (up to 102°F) and malaise (that achy, "blah" feeling we all associate with the flu). The prostate gland itself may feel swollen and rigid when your doctor examines you and may be extremely sensitive to touch or pressure. The swelling may choke off the flow of urine to the point that urination becomes extremely difficult or even impossible. In most cases, microscopic examination of a urine specimen reveals pus and bacteriuria.

Chronic bacterial prostatitis, characterized by recurrent bacteriuria, is relatively uncommon.

Q: How is bacterial prostatitis treated?

A: Acute bacterial prostatitis can be treated with one of several oral antibiotics, depending on the bacterial species identified in the urine. Symptoms of acute bacterial prostatitis often resolve quickly with antibacterial therapy, but treatment is typically continued for several weeks to ensure that residual bacteria are eliminated. In a particularly severe case, when high fever occurs or when the swelling of the prostate constricts the urethra to the point that urination is impossible, the man is usually hospitalized for insertion of a catheter to drain the bladder and for treatment with intravenous antibiotics.

Chronic bacterial prostatitis is less responsive to antibiotics than acute prostatitis and may require a course of treatment lasting up to 12 weeks.

Prostate Cancer

Q: What about prostate cancer? How serious is it?

A: In the United States, cancer of the prostate is the most common form of cancer affecting men and is second only to lung cancer as a cause of cancer death among men. Each year, more than 130,000 men in this country are diagnosed with prostatic cancer. And each year, more than 30,000 die from it.

Prostate cancer is rare in men younger than 50 years of age, but the incidence increases with age. Assuming a life expectancy of 75 years, 42 percent of men will develop prostatic cancer by age 75. Prostate cancer is responsible for nearly 3 percent of all deaths of men over age 55. Family history of prostate cancer is a known risk factor. In addition, African-American men are twice as likely as white men to develop prostate cancer.

Q: What are the symptoms of prostate cancer, and how is it diagnosed?

A: Many times there are no symptoms, even in the latter stages of disease; however, when symptoms are present, they may include dysuria (painful urination), increased frequency of urination, back or hip pain or blood in the urine.

The most useful technique for diagnosis is a **digital rectal exam (DRE)**, during which the doctor inserts a lubricated, gloved finger into the rectum and feels the prostate gland. In addition, there are biochemical markers for prostate cancer that can be detected by laboratory tests; of these, the most sensitive is a test that measures blood levels of a substance called **prostate-specific antigen (PSA)**. Various forms of diagnostic imaging may also be employed, including ultrasound, magnetic resonance imaging (MRI) and computed tomography (CT). Biopsy of the prostate—the removal of a small sample of prostate tissue—is also necessary to confirm the diagnosis.

Q: How is prostate cancer treated?

A: It depends on how advanced the cancer is. Surgical removal of the prostate (prostatectomy) is the oldest form of treatment. Radiation therapy is an acceptable alternative for some men. Another mode of treatment involves suppressing the production of male hormones (androgens), which control the growth of the prostate. This can be accomplished by removing the testes and the adrenal glands, both of which produce androgens, or by antagonizing androgen production by giving the man female hormones (estrogens). A final option is chemotherapy with anticancer drugs—usually reserved for patients with very advanced disease that has spread to other sites in the body. Nontreatment should also be considered. Prostate cancer grows very slowly, so some men may want to forgo treatment altogether if the cancer is limited.

Q: I've heard that removal of the prostate results in impotence and **incontinence**—is that true?

A: That was more true in the past than today. Thanks to refinements in surgical technique, most men who undergo prostatectomy are not left with erectile dysfunction (ED). The risk of incontinence (inability to control when urination occurs) is between 1 and 4 percent. ED is more of a problem after radiation therapy, affecting 30 to 60 percent of patients, depending on the technique employed.

Q: Can prostate cancer be prevented?

A: We don't know how to prevent prostate cancer, but as is the case with other cancers, early detection is the next best thing. The American Cancer Society recommends that all men over 50 years of age have a PSA test and DRE every year.

Peyronie's Disease

Q: What is Peyronie's disease?

A: Peyronie's disease is a condition that causes the erect penis to bend to one side. As described in chapter 2, there are two side-by-side chambers of erectile tissue in the penis called the corpora cavernosa. In Peyronie's disease, one of the corpus cavernosa becomes weakened by the adjacent growth of fibrous tissue. During erection, the penis bends toward the side with the fibrous growth. It can be painful and embarrassing and can interfere with penetration and ejaculation.

Q: What causes the fibrous tissue in Peyronie's disease? How is the condition treated?

A: Trauma to the penis and urethritis may contribute to the development of Peyronie's disease, but these connections are speculative. The truth is that we don't really know what causes it, how to treat it or how to avoid it. If necessary, uncomplicated cases often can be corrected with surgery. Though hardly a common problem, the incidence of Peyronie's disease is thought by some to be on the rise.

Epididymitis

Q: What is epididymitis?

A: As we described in chapter 2, attached to each testis is a coiled tube, called the epididymis, in which sperm cells mature. Epididymitis is the inflammation of this tube and usually affects only one testis at a time. It may cause the scrotum to become red and swollen, and because it can be so painful, it has been called "great balls of fire." Other symptoms include fever and urethritis.

Q: What causes epididymitis, and how is it treated?

A: Seventy percent of cases in heterosexual men younger than 35 years of age are caused by chlamydia, and most of the remainder are attributed to gonorrhea.

In homosexual men, the most likely cause is bacterial infection acquired through anal intercourse. Because different pathogens are involved, urethritis is rare in such cases, though bacteriuria is common.

Antibiotic therapy is standard for epididymitis. The condition can result in permanent sterility if left untreated.

Orchitis

Q: What is orchitis?

A: In medical terminology, the prefix *orchi* refers to the testes, and *itis* designates inflammation, so orchitis is inflammation of one or both testes. It sometimes accompanies acute bacterial prostatitis, inflammation of the seminal vesicles (glands that secrete about 60 percent of the component fluid of semen) and a handful of other conditions. Most commonly, however, orchitis is a complication of postchildhood mumps, occurring in 20 to 30 percent of cases. Mumps orchitis is also the most troublesome form of orchitis.

Q: What are the signs and symptoms of orchitis, and how is it treated?

A: Signs and symptoms include malaise, headache, nausea and vomiting. Shaking chills are common, as is high fever (103°F to 106°F). The affected testis becomes quite swollen and painful, and the epididymis can be felt through the scrotum—swollen and cordlike.

There is no specific treatment available for mumps or mumps orchitis. Corticosteroids are often given for fever and symptomatic relief of mumps orchitis. In about 50 percent of cases, a testis affected by mumps orchitis will waste away after the inflammation subsides.

Q: I always heard that if you got mumps after childhood, it would leave you sterile. Is this true?

A: Not in all cases. If only one testis is affected, the man still has the other testis. If both are affected and both atrophy, however, he will probably be left with low sperm count or complete sterility.

Testicular Cancer

Q: How widespread a problem is testicular cancer?

A: Testicular cancer is not all that common. Each year, roughly three out of every 100,000 men develop testicular cancer. African-American men have substantially lower rates than whites (0.9 per 100,000 men, compared with 3 per 100,000 for whites), but we don't know why. The total number of new cases per year in the United States is estimated at between 5,500 and 6,000. Despite these low numbers, you should know that testicular cancer is the most common form of cancer affecting men between the ages of 15 and 35. Statistically, the chances of developing testicular cancer are greatest between the ages of 20 and 40. Testicular cancer is quite rare between the ages of 40 and 60, after which the risk begins to rise again. Between 2 and 3 percent of cases involve both testes, either simultaneously or one after the other.

Q: Are there any risk factors for testicular cancer?

A: Men with a history of **undescended testis**, also known as **cryptorchism**, have three to 14 times higher rates of testicular cancer than men without such a history. (With undescended testis, the organ does not descend from the abdomen into the scrotum just after birth as it should.) Between 5 and 10 percent of men with a history of cryptorchism in one testis develop cancer in the other testis. The reason is not known.

Q: How serious is testicular cancer? Can it be cured?

A: Any form of cancer is serious, but the good news is that testicular cancer has one of the highest cure rates of any solid tumor. In fact, testicular cancer is often held up as a model for the modern treatment of solid tumors. As recently as the 1970s, only 10 percent of testicular cancer patients survived the disease. Today, the overall survival rate is 90 percent. There are several types of testicular cancer, and depending on the type and how far the cancer has progressed before it is detected and treated, cure rates may be as high as 100 percent.

Q: What are the signs and symptoms of testicular cancer?

A: Men most often come to the doctor complaining of a painless swelling or nodule in one testis. It is usually described as a lump or hardness and is sometimes accompanied by a sensation of heaviness or a dull ache in the lower abdomen or scrotum. About 10 percent of men with testicular cancer have severe pain. Sometimes a fertility problem is the symptom that alerts the doctor to testicular cancer.

Roughly 10 percent of men with testicular cancer experience signs and symptoms related to the spread of the cancer to other organs and systems. These may take the form of a lump in the neck, breathing difficulties, gastrointestinal problems or lower back pain. Five percent of men with the most common type of testicular cancer experience breast enlargement.

Q: How is testicular cancer diagnosed and treated?

A: Any firm, solid mass or lump found in a testis is assumed to be testicular cancer. The doctor will then attempt to rule out other conditions and diseases that can mimic testicular cancer. If these other conditions cannot be ruled out, the next step is to remove the affected testis—a procedure known as **orchiectomy**.

The removed testis is then carefully examined to determine the type of testicular cancer and to determine if it is confined to the testis. If there is evidence that the tumor has started to spread beyond the confines of the testis, it may also be necessary to remove the lymph nodes nearest to the testes. Beyond surgical removal of the affected testis and nearby lymph nodes, therapy for testicular cancer generally involves a combination of measures. Therapy depends on the type and stage of disease—the more advanced the disease, the more complex the treatment—and may include radiation therapy and chemotherapy with anticancer drugs.

Q: Can testicular cancer be prevented?

A: We don't know how to prevent testicular cancer. However, the next best thing to prevention is early detection, and the key to early detection is **testicular self-examination**—a procedure whereby you regularly and frequently examine your own testes for signs of cancer. As described below, it's a simple, two-minute procedure a man can do after a shower. Turn it into a habit, and it could save your life.

It's worth noting that 95 percent of testicular cancer is of a type called germ cell tumor, and survival with this type is directly related to how far the disease has progressed by the time treatment is initiated. A delay of one to two months between the earliest detectable phases of disease and the actual clinical diagnosis by a physician is all too common.

The American Medical Association recommends that you routinely examine your testes once a week, using the following procedure. Again, perform this examination after your shower or bath, when the scrotum is relaxed.

- Hold each testis with both hands and gently roll it between your fingers and thumb.
- Gently feel the surface of each testis for a lump or swelling.
- Spend 30 to 60 seconds on each testis.
- If you find a lump or notice any kind of swelling, contact your doctor immediately.

Other Testicular Problems

Q: Earlier, you mentioned testicular torsion. Is it related to testicular cancer?

A: No, it's actually more of a mechanical problem. Testicular torsion describes what happens when one of the testes becomes twisted out of its normal position inside the scrotum. It can result in the kinking of blood vessels, which shuts down blood flow to and from the testis. Testicular torsion is not a common condition, but when it occurs, it most often affects adolescents. The chief symptom is sudden pain in the affected testis followed by swelling, redness and tenderness of the scrotum. The pain can indeed be agonizing—bad enough to cause nausea and vomiting.

Q: How is testicular torsion treated?

A: Some cases resolve on their own, without medical intervention. When this happens, relief from pain and swelling is immediate. Unresolved cases demand immediate medical attention. Sometimes the testis can be restored to its normal position by gentle manipulation; if not, surgery is required. Failure to seek immediate attention may result in the loss of the testis if it is severely damaged or if blood flow has been interrupted for a prolonged period of time.

Q: What is a hydrocele?

A: Within the scrotum, each testis is surrounded by membranes containing fluid that allows for the well-lubricated movement of the testis. Sometimes, for reasons unknown, an excess of this fluid begins to collect between the testis and the membranes, causing the scrotum to swell. This accumulation of fluid is called a hydrocele.

Q: It sounds painful. How is it treated?

A: Small hydroceles generally are not painful and do not require medical intervention. If the hydrocele becomes large and painful, the excess fluid can be drained off with a hypodermic needle and a syringe under a local anesthetic. Recurrent cases sometimes require surgery to tighten the membranous covering of the testis.

Q: Is hydrocele a common phenomenon, and is it serious?

A: Hydrocele is common, especially among older men, and although hydroceles are harmless, any swelling of the testes should be checked out by your doctor to rule out other, more serious diseases and conditions.

5 CONTRACEPTION AND FERTILITY

Q: Fertility and contraception are sort of opposite concepts, aren't they? It seems odd to discuss them here together.

A: Not necessarily. In the larger context of sexual health, we see them as different folds in the same cloth. Fertility—the ability to become pregnant and give birth—is our natural biological condition. It allows us to reproduce, ensuring the survival of our species. But our fertility is expressed through a powerful sexuality, and the natural consequences of sexual activity are not always in our best interests. The spread of STDs is one area where this is true. Unwanted pregnancy is another.

Contraception, in a sense, represents our triumph over biology. Safe, effective methods of birth control allow us to manage our fertility to the greater benefit of the individual *and* society. Contraception allows us to fully experience our sexuality while choosing if and when to have a child. It allows us to plan our lives more rationally and to keep our domestic needs in scale with our economic and personal resources. Reproductive science has also made great strides against infertility—the inability to conceive and give birth—satisfying the reproductive needs of many whose fertility is in some way impaired.

But before we get into the details of contraception and fertility, let's take another look at human reproduction and the mechanics of **conception**.

CONCEPTION

Q: When does conception occur?

A: Conception begins with **fertilization**—the union of an **ovum**, or egg, from the woman and a sperm from the man. The egg and the sperm each have half the genetic material needed to make a human being. Together, they have the potential to make a new whole.

At risk of repeating a lesson in the birds and the bees, here's how fertilization occurs: When no contraceptive is used, sperm cells deposited in the vagina can swim up through the uterus and into the woman's fallopian tubes where they may find an egg. The sperm cells are programmed to search for and attempt to penetrate (fertilize) an egg. When just one sperm succeeds in this task, fertilization has occurred. The egg then surrounds itself with a protective cover so no other sperm may enter. The fertilized egg continues moving down the fallopian tube to the uterus where it becomes embedded in the wall of the uterus. There, nourished by blood, it continues to grow. And if all goes well, the woman gives birth to a baby in approximately nine months.

Q: You've already mentioned that sperm come from the testes. Where does the egg come from?

A: A woman produces and develops eggs in her ovaries, and she has all the eggs she's ever going to have on the day she is born—as many as 200,000 immature eggs in each ovary.

Mature human eggs are spherical in shape and measure 0.07 to 0.17 millimeter in diameter; they are, in fact, the largest cells in the human body and are visible to the naked eye. Once a month, a woman ovulates—that is, one of her ovaries releases a mature egg, which travels down her fallopian tube toward the uterus. As this happens, the wall of the uterus becomes enriched with blood and tissue in preparation to receive a fertilized egg.

Q: When does a woman ovulate?

A: A woman's menstrual cycle averages 28 days. This can vary from woman to woman and from one cycle to the next in the same woman. Many factors can affect the *length* of the entire menstrual cycle, but ovulation generally occurs approximately *14 days before* the onset of menstrual flow. Most women have no physical sensation when ovulation occurs, but there are subtle physical changes that can be detected by a number of methods that we explain later in this chapter.

CONTRACEPTION AND FERTILITY 139

Q: What happens to the egg when a woman doesn't conceive a child?

A: If no fertilized egg is received, the woman has her normal monthly period, during which the blood that has built up to nourish the fertilized egg drains from the uterus along with the egg.

Q: Can a small amount of semen result in conception?

A: Yes. Technically, it takes only one sperm to fertilize an egg. On the other hand, the odds of any single sperm reaching the egg are pretty low—literally one in a million. A typical ejaculation produces about a teaspoon of semen containing between 200 million and 400 million sperm, but only 200 to 400 ever reach the fallopian tube bearing the egg.

Q: What are the odds that one act of vaginal intercourse will result in conception?

A: That depends on many factors, but the chief factor is the time in the menstrual cycle when the act of intercourse occurs. Published research would say that the "relative risk" of conception from one act of unprotected intercourse ranges from roughly zero on day one of the menstrual cycle to about one in four on the day before ovulation.

Q: How long do sperm survive in the woman's body?

A: Sperm can survive in a woman's uterus and fallopian tubes for up to one week, but more typically they survive about three days, or 72 hours.

CONTRACEPTION

Q: Now that I understand how fertilization and conception occur, let's talk about how to prevent it. How do the different birth control methods work? Do they mainly kill sperm?

A: Contraception generally means one of two things: ensuring that a sperm cell does not fertilize an egg or ensuring that a fertilized egg does not become implanted in the wall of the uterus.

Methods fall generally into two categories. Some are considered reversible—that is, they do not affect a person's long-term fertility. Others are considered irreversible, or essentially permanent.

Reversible methods include the following:

- *Barrier methods.* These include condoms, diaphragms and **cervical caps**, all of which create a physical or chemical barrier between sperm and egg. The chemical barrier we mention is spermicide, a detergentlike compound that destroys sperm by breaking down the membrane of the surface of sperm cells.

- *Intrauterine devices (IUDs).* These have been said to prevent conception by preventing the implantation of a fertilized egg, but the latest research suggests that they work primarily by preventing fertilization.

- *Hormonal methods.* The birth control pill, hormonal injections and hormonal implants are also reversible. These forms of contraception work by preventing ovulation.

Techniques that may not be reversible include **tubal ligation** and **vasectomy**; both are also referred to as **sterilization**. These procedures are surgical. Tubal ligation closes off the fallopian tube, preventing the egg from entering the uterus. Vasectomy cuts the vas deferens, preventing sperm from mixing with the semen. Occasionally, these surgical methods may be reversed, but they should generally be seen as permanent measures.

Q: How do I choose the best method of birth control?

A: Important issues to consider are the safety and effectiveness of the method; its cost and availability; whether it interrupts or interferes with your sexual pleasure; whether you are also seeking protection against sexually transmitted diseases (STDs); and how much personal control the method requires.

No single method of birth control is appropriate for everyone. In fact, it's often true that a person or couple will change methods of contraception over time, depending on changes in the status of the relationship or other health considerations. What is most important is that individuals or couples choose a method of birth control that they will use properly and consistently.

Q: How do I know a method of contraception is effective? How is this determined?

A: When researchers look at the effectiveness of a particular method of contraception, they weigh two factors: the effectiveness of the method when used perfectly—under highly supervised and controlled conditions—and the effectiveness of the method in typical, everyday use. For example, with a hormonal implant, there is no difference between perfect use and typical use; once implanted, it simply does its job. On the other hand, with an unreliable method such as **withdrawal** (removing the penis from the vagina before ejaculation), the difference between perfect use and typical use is quite high. Many times, the effectiveness of a method is expressed as a percentage. The rate of effectiveness is essentially the percentage of women who don't get pregnant with use; the failure rate is the percentage of women who do get pregnant with use. When considering a method of birth control, you need to understand not just its theoretical effectiveness with perfect use but also the potential for misuse or incorrect use and whether you are likely to be a "perfect" practitioner of the method.

Oral Contraceptives

Q: Let's talk about specific forms of contraception. How does the birth control pill work?

A: Birth control pills, also known as **oral contraceptives**, contain a synthetic combination of the hormones estrogen and progesterone, both of which are instrumental in preparing the female reproductive tract to conceive and carry a baby. (Progesterone-only pills are also available, though they are generally less effective than the combination.)

The Pill provides a daily dose of hormones that prevent ovulation and change the cervical mucus and lining of the uterus to interfere with conception. The Pill is a widely utilized form of contraception in the United States. Of all the women in this country who use some form of contraception, 31 percent rely on the Pill.

Q: How effective is the Pill in preventing pregnancy?

A: By almost any measure, very effective. In the perfect-use scenario, only one out of 1,000 women (0.1 percent) would become pregnant during the first year of use. However, in typical, "real world" use, an average of five women out of 100 (5 percent) become pregnant during their first year on the Pill. These pregnancies most commonly occur because of a lack of consistency in taking the drug or because women discontinue the Pill without having a backup method in place.

Q: What are the advantages and disadvantages of oral contraceptives?

A: The benefits of the Pill are that it is safe, effective and easy to use and does not interfere with a couple's sexual pleasure. It can be used for many years without reducing fertility, and it carries health benefits such as menstrual regularity and reduced risk of cancers and ovarian cysts. Studies show that a woman using the Pill for up to four years is 30 percent less likely to develop ovarian cancer, and the risk continues to decline with extended use. The numbers are similar for endometrial cancer.

The disadvantages are that the Pill has to be taken daily and may be expensive for some (about $200 a year plus a visit to a clinic or doctor's office). In addition, possible side effects include nausea, headaches and decreased sexual appetite. Equally important, the Pill does not prevent the transmission of STDs.

While considered a safe enough method to be under consideration for over-the-counter availability, studies of the Pill suggest some long-term risks. These include a slightly increased risk of circulatory system diseases such as stroke and thrombosis (blood clots in the leg). However, the risk of such problems from the Pill is less significant than the risk from other factors such as obesity, diabetes and smoking. The effect of oral contraceptives on breast cancer is still a matter of study. According to an analysis in the 1998 edition of *Contraceptive Technology*, the rate of breast cancer may be 24 percent higher in women who currently use the Pill than in nonusers, but this drops markedly for each year that women are off the Pill.

Intrauterine Devices

Q: What is an intrauterine device?

A: An intrauterine device (IUD) is a small, usually T-shaped plastic rod that contains either copper or progesterone. An IUD must be inserted into the uterus by a doctor or other health care provider. The device has a string that hangs through the cervix into the vagina so that the woman can check to see if the device is properly in place.

Though IUDs have been used for many years—similar devices, in fact, were employed in ancient times—scientists do not know precisely how IUDs work. It was once believed that this foreign body created an inflammatory reaction in the uterus that prevented the fertilized egg from implanting in the uterine wall. More recent data suggest that the IUD causes an increase in specific uterine and tubal fluids that block fertilization.

Depending on the type of device, an IUD can remain in the uterus from one to 10 years. Removal of the IUD must be carried out by a doctor or other properly trained health care provider.

Q: Weren't IUDs taken off the market at one time? Are they safe?

A: A number of IUDs have been taken off the U.S. market over the last three decades. By far the most well-publicized of these cases was the 1974 recall of the Dalkon Shield, manufactured by A.H. Robins, because it was linked with increased risk of pregnancy complications and pelvic inflammatory disease. Subsequent research suggested that many of the problems associated with this IUD could be traced to infection at the time of insertion or to sexually transmitted diseases such as chlamydia. In any case, the two redesigned IUDs on the U.S. market today—the copper T and progesterone T—are considered safe and effective.

Q: How effective is the IUD in preventing pregnancy?

A: The IUD that uses copper has a failure rate of less than 1 percent—rivaling surgical sterilization for effectiveness—and the progesterone-based IUD has a failure rate of less than 2 percent—a figure slightly better than the Pill. Since the device is inserted by a health care provider and remains in place, there is no difference between perfect and typical use.

Q: What are the advantages and disadvantages of the IUD?

A: On the positive side, the IUD is ready when you are. It requires no interruption in the natural flow of sexual events (like stopping to put on a condom does). And since it does not require the user to take any regular action, there is no potential for error. IUDs can remain in the body for several years, but the contraceptive effect is gone once the IUD is removed. There is no residual effect.

The disadvantages: IUDs can lead to increased menstrual cramps and excessive menstrual bleeding in some women. Like the Pill, the IUD also offers no protection against STDs and may increase the risk of PID, which can lead to infertility or sterility, shortly after insertion. In addition, an IUD must be removed immediately in the rare instance that a woman becomes pregnant.

The method is considered most appropriate for women who have only one partner, who have no other risk factors for PID and who have already given birth. Insertion of an IUD, which can be uncomfortable, requires a visit to the clinic or doctor's office and costs between $300 and $400.

Implants and Injectables

Q: What about injectable and implanted contraceptives? How do they work?

A: There are two main forms of contraception that are either injected into or implanted in the body; respectively, they are medroxyprogesterone acetate suspension (**Depo-Provera**) and levonorgestrel (**Norplant**).

Depo-Provera, the only injectable contraceptive available in the

United States, is a synthetic progesterone injected into a woman's arm or buttocks every three months. The progesterone hinders ovulation and thickens the cervical mucus, making it harder for the sperm to enter the uterus. Progesterone also makes it difficult for the fertilized egg to implant in the wall of the uterus.

Norplant consists of six matchstick-size silicone cylinders that are surgically implanted under the skin of a woman's upper arm. Progesterone from the implant is released for up to five years, causing the same contraceptive action that it does in Depo-Provera. The implants must be surgically removed.

Q: How effective are the injectable and implanted contraceptives?

A: Depo-Provera and Norplant are both highly effective forms of birth control. Since they are both long-term methods administered by a clinician, there is no difference between typical and perfect use. The average failure rate for both is less than 1 percent. Of women using Depo-Provera, only three of every 1,000 women (0.3 percent) become pregnant in the first year of use. For Norplant, the number is one of every 2,000 (0.05 percent), although Norplant is somewhat less effective over time. Over a five-year period, 1.8 of every 100 (1.8 percent) women using Norplant become pregnant.

Q: What are the advantages and disadvantages of injectable and implanted contraceptives?

A: Both Depo-Provera and Norplant are effective, long-lasting birth control methods that are reversible. They eliminate the potential for user error, do not disrupt or interfere with sexual intercourse and are particularly appealing for those who find taking a daily pill difficult. Both reduce menstrual cramps and appear to help decrease incidences of PID, endometrial cancer and ovarian cancer.

The main disadvantage of these methods is disruption of the menstrual cycle. Some women will have more than their average number of days of light bleeding, while others may find that their periods stop altogether—*not* an unwelcome change for many women. Progesterone-based contraception can also cause weight gain and breast tenderness in some women. And neither of these two methods offers protection against STDs. Lastly, Depo-Provera may delay a return to fertility for six to 12 months.

Both methods require a visit to a clinic or doctor's office. Depo-Provera requires a visit to a clinic every 12 weeks. Each injection costs about $35 ($140 a year), in addition to the cost of the office visits. Norplant requires minor surgery, which usually costs between $500 and $700, including the cost of insertion and removal. Over the course of five years, this comes out to $100 to $150 per year.

Q: So far, all these birth control methods seem to focus on the woman's body! Are there any other options that focus on the man?

A: Researchers have tried for years to develop a birth control pill for men, but there have always been drawbacks such as toxicity, erectile dysfunction and long-term infertility. Research continues, however. A small study done in 1996 got very promising results and very few side effects with a combination of oral testosterone and progestin.

Studies are also being conducted on injectable contraceptives for men, which involve various combinations of hormones that either reduce sperm count or render sperm temporarily ineffective.

More research is needed on all of these methods, none of which is yet available in the United States. As a result, most men rely on condoms when they take responsibility for birth control.

Male Condoms

Q: Are condoms still a viable contraceptive option? How exactly do they prevent pregnancy?

A: The male condom is a sheath of latex, polyurethane or a natural membrane that fits over the erect penis to prevent semen from entering a woman's vagina during intercourse and to prevent the spread of STDs. As we explained in chapter 3, the condom must be rolled down over the penis when the penis is erect and before intercourse begins. After intercourse, the man must withdraw from the woman while his penis is still erect and then remove the condom. Each condom should be used only once. See chapter 3 for more information on proper use of condoms as protection against STDs.

When used properly, the traditional male condom is an effective method of birth control, used by roughly 14 percent of couples employing contraception, and it offers excellent protection against many STDs.

Q: So how effective is the condom in preventing pregnancy?

A: With perfect use, condoms fail to prevent pregnancy only 3 percent of the time—about the same rate as the Pill. However, the failure rate for typical condom use is 14 percent, reflecting the fact that mistakes can be made in using this method.

Q: What are the advantages and disadvantages of the condom?

A: Condoms are one of the least expensive methods, are easy to use and are readily available over the counter. The average condom costs a little less than $1, so a couple who has sex twice a week using condoms will spend about $100 per year on contraception. Further, condoms allow the man to take an active part in pregnancy prevention. They have no side effects except for the potential to cause skin irritation (and in rare cases, a severe systemic reaction) in those allergic to latex. And of course, by comparison with any other method of birth control, condoms offer excellent protection against HIV and many other STDs.

The chief disadvantage with condoms is that they must be properly put on and taken off to be effective, and many couples do not reliably use them for every sexual contact. A second issue is breakage or slippage. Condoms also require a high degree of personal responsibility. Sexual activity must be interrupted or modified to put on a condom, and many men complain of a loss of sexual sensitivity—an important barrier to condom use. This loss of sensation can be marked enough to interfere with orgasm for men and to increase the risk of slippage due to a waning erection. Interestingly, some women also report complaints such as condom discomfort during intercourse.

Q: How often do condoms break or slip?

A: Not as often as is sometimes rumored. Studies show rates as high as 7 percent for breakage during vaginal intercourse or withdrawal, but the average is about 2 percent. Slippage is actually a more common problem. Researchers calculate that condoms fall off the penis entirely in 1 to 5 percent of acts of vaginal intercourse and may slip down the penis twice that often.

Breakage and slippage rates during anal intercourse are probably higher, and new condoms specifically for anal sex are being designed and marketed in Europe.

Incidentally, condoms are regulated by the Food and Drug Administration (FDA) as a medical device, and every manufacturer must test each batch of its product electronically for holes and weak spots before it is shipped to market.

Q: Are some condoms better than others?

A: As we mentioned before, the traditional condom is currently available in three different materials: natural membrane, latex and polyurethane.

Natural-membrane condoms have been used for contraception and disease prevention for many decades, and they have their loyal users despite being the most expensive option of the three. During the 1980s, however, research showed that microscopic pores in these condoms were actually larger than some of the sexually transmitted viruses, such as hepatitis B and HIV. For this reason, public health officials began to specify use of latex condoms in their efforts to stop the spread of HIV and other STDs.

The latex condom is the least expensive and most popular of the three types. It is available in various colors and textures, both with and without lubrication and with and without spermicide.

Polyurethane condoms have been on the market since the mid-1990s. They conduct heat better than latex and thus offer greater sensation to users, but they have been shown to have higher slippage and breakage rates. The polyurethane condom is a good option for men and women allergic to latex.

There are other differences among condoms as well, in that some are prelubricated and some not; some are colored, flavored or ribbed; and some have a nipplelike reservoir at the tip to collect semen. Research on consumer preferences has shown that few men care about color and other novelty features but do prefer condoms that are prelubricated and have the reservoir tip.

Vaginal Barriers

Q: Can you tell me about the **female condom**. How does it work?

A: The female condom (also known as the vaginal pouch) is a cylinder of thin polyurethane about six inches long and two inches wide, with one open end and one closed end—each reinforced by a flexible plastic ring.

The closed end, with its smaller ring, is inserted into the vagina and fitted over the cervix. The open end with the larger ring sits just outside the vaginal lips. Positioned in this way, the female condom prevents sperm from entering the vagina and also helps protect against STDs. It does not require spermicide to achieve this dual protection. Like the male condom, the female condom is designed for single use only.

Q: How effective is the female condom at preventing pregnancy?

A: The female condom is relatively new, and research is still underway to determine its effectiveness in typical use. With perfect use, the female condom fails only 5 percent of the time, but the failure rate in typical use is estimated at 21 percent, largely because proper insertion requires more skill than most other methods.

Q: What are the advantages and disadvantages of the female condom?

A: The female condom puts the woman in control of contraception. It's available over the counter and offers a combination of contraception and STD protection. But its novelty is one of its disadvantages. Few women understand it or know how to use it properly. Some are put off by its size and look or by the squeaking noise it sometimes makes during intercourse. The female condom is also more expensive than the male condom—costing between $3 and $5 each.

As regards sensation, some users believe it is superior to the male condom and may provide a degree of clitoral stimulation. Others report that it reduces sensation for both partners.

Q: How is a diaphragm, another sort of vaginal barrier, different from a female condom?

A: One major difference is that the diaphragm, unlike most other vaginal barrier methods, relies on spermicide for effectiveness.

The diaphragm, a barrier device that prevents sperm from entering the uterus, is a rubber dome with a thick, flexible rim that fits into the vagina and covers the cervix. A woman must go to a doctor or clinician to obtain a diaphragm that fits properly. The device can be put in place up to six hours before intercourse. It is covered with a spermicidal jelly or cream and then inserted into the vagina so it fits over the cervix.

Because the spermicide is critical to effectiveness, it should be reapplied to the device if the couple engages in a second or third—or tenth!—act of vaginal intercourse more than six hours after the first application. For the same reason, a diaphragm should not be removed until six to eight hours after the last act of intercourse. (It should not, however, be left in place for more than 24 hours, a practice that can cause sores and possibly create a risk of toxic shock syndrome, a potentially deadly infection.)

Q: How effective is the diaphragm in preventing pregnancy?

A: With perfect use, 6 percent of women become pregnant using the diaphragm. With typical use, the number rises to 20 percent.

Q: What are the advantages and disadvantages of the diaphragm?

A: Unlike other barrier methods of contraception, the diaphragm does not interrupt sexual activity, does not decrease sensitivity during sex and has very few potential side effects. The cost ranges from $50 to $150, depending on the charge for the clinic visit.

Some women find the diaphragm hard to insert. Initially, a woman must go to a clinic to have the diaphragm fitted, and she needs to have it checked regularly and possibly changed every couple of years. Further, the diaphragm may increase the risk of urinary tract infections if it is too large. Occasionally, it can become dislodged during sex, compromising its contraceptive effectiveness. Lastly, it's uncertain whether the device offers substantial protection against STDs.

Q: How does a cervical cap differ from the diaphragm? How does it work?

A: The cervical cap is similar to the diaphragm in concept. It is a thimble-shaped piece of latex that fits over the cervix and prevents sperm from entering the uterus. Like a diaphragm, the cervical cap must be used in combination with a spermicide. And as with the diaphragm, a woman must go to a clinic or doctor's office to be fitted.

Q: How effective is the cervical cap?

A: With perfect use, 9 percent of women become pregnant with the cervical cap. With typical use, the number rises to 20 percent. After a woman has been pregnant, however, the effectiveness of the cervical cap drops markedly: The failure rate increases to 26 percent with perfect use and 40 percent with typical use—unacceptably high for many users.

Q: What are the advantages and disadvantages of the cervical cap?

A: The advantages and disadvantages are similar to those of the diaphragm. The cervical cap fits more tightly than a diaphragm, but it can also be more difficult to remove. The cost ranges from $50 to $150, depending on the charge for the office visit. It should be replaced yearly.

Natural Methods

Q: What if I want to use a natural method of contraception? What are my options?

A: The most well-known natural contraceptive method is the rhythm method. The rhythm method, or calendar method, refers to the practice of abstaining from vaginal sex each month around the time of a woman's peak fertility. Specifically, the rhythm method charts the average length of a woman's menstrual cycle, then attempts to predict when ovulation will take place. This calculation involves the three following probabilities.

- Ovulation usually occurs on the fourteenth day.
- An egg lives one day after ovulation.
- Sperm can live up to a week inside a woman's body, but typically last 72 hours, or three days.

Based on these probabilities, a couple will not conceive if they abstain from sex between the ninth and the sixteenth day of the cycle. (Two days are added to safeguard against late ovulation.)

Q: How can a woman tell more precisely when she's ovulating?

A: As a variation on the calendar method, many women use what are called **fertility awareness methods**. They include the basal body temperature method and the cervical mucus method.

The basal body temperature method depends on a woman charting the temperature of her body first thing in the morning and marking the rise in temperature that normally occurs during and after ovulation. To do this properly, she needs to use a basal thermometer, which is calibrated differently from a normal fever thermometer in order to highlight small variations in temperature. Careful recordkeeping over a period of several months often reveals a consistent pattern of ovulation on a particular day in the menstrual cycle.

With the mucus method, a woman monitors changes in cervical mucus that occur around the time of ovulation. The mucus method requires that a woman use either her fingers or toilet tissue to collect a sample of fluid from the vaginal opening. The sample is judged for wetness, elasticity and other characteristics. In general, the likelihood of ovulation increases when mucus becomes both abundant and elastic, sometimes comparable to the consistency of raw egg white. Immediately after ovulation, the mucus becomes tacky.

The mucus method requires some subjective judgments, to be sure, but some women find that with instruction and practice they can observe a very definite pattern that helps to predict ovulation.

Q: Are there other options? Can you combine these methods?

A: Yes. The symptothermal method is a combination of the above strategies and has been shown to be a slightly better predictor than either the cervical mucus or basal body temperature method used alone.

Also, some women experience a marked lower abdominal pain or cramping around the time of ovulation. This is known as Mittelschmertz, German for "middle pain." In addition, home test kits that attempt to predict ovulation based on hormone levels are available over the counter, but the accuracy of these has not been well studied.

Q: How effective are fertility awareness methods of birth control, and are they considered good contraceptive options?

A: Fertility awareness methods rely entirely on a couple being able to track the woman's fertility and to abstain from sex during the period of possible conception. If done correctly, they can be very effective—more effective than various barrier methods. In perfect practice, these methods have a failure rate of 1 to 9 percent, depending on the type of method. However, in the real world, 13 to 20 percent of couples who rely on fertility awareness methods become pregnant in the first year. The most effective adaptation of these methods is to have sex only after ovulation has taken place and the egg is no longer viable, which means ruling out vaginal sex for half the month.

There are advantages to these methods, however. For one, they are the only methods available to strict adherents of certain religions. Cost is negligible (the price of a thermometer), and there are no side effects. As disadvantages, there is no STD protection and the method requires persistent effort. Nonetheless, for motivated couples, it is a viable option.

Q: Is it true that breastfeeding acts as a natural contraceptive?

A: Partially, yes. When a woman nurses, her body produces prolactin, a hormone that suppresses ovulation. This contraceptive effect, however, is tied to a certain frequency of breastfeeding—a feeding every four hours during the day and every six hours at night and very little supplementation with formula. Also, there is no efficient way to predict when the level of prolactin will fall enough to allow renewed ovulation. In other words, the problem with relying on breastfeeding is that a couple may not know ovulation has resumed until after the woman is pregnant again. (The woman would not have begun menstruating until after she ovulated, and that would be too late.) On the other hand, this method is usually effective for six months postpartum and possibly for as long as 12 months if full breastfeeding continues.

Emergency Contraception

Q: I've been hearing a lot about emergency contraception, or **morning-after contraception**, recently. What exactly is it?

A: Morning-after contraception refers to techniques that prevent a fertilized egg from implanting in the uterus. There are two types of emergency contraception—**morning-after pills** and the IUD—either of which can be used in an emergency such as when a condom breaks or a diaphragm becomes dislodged. Neither is considered an option for everyday use. The pills are only 75 percent effective and cause severe side effects such as nausea, vomiting and short-term alterations of the menstrual cycle.

Most morning-after pills contain high doses of synthetic estrogen. One dose is taken as soon as possible after intercourse, and a second dose follows 12 hours after the first. These pills are most effective if dosing is completed between 12 and 24 hours after unprotected sex or contraceptive failure. They are ineffective if given after 72 hours. An alternative regimen using levonogestrel alone is under development, and it has been shown to have lower pregnancy rates and fewer side effects.

Other medications are often given along with the pills to prevent the side effect of vomiting, which may purge the contraceptive medication if it occurs. Some women experience headaches, dizziness and abdominal cramping. These side effects go away a couple of days after the final treatment.

An IUD can also be used for emergency contraception. The device is inserted within five to seven days after unprotected intercourse. Though it has a very low failure rate, this option is used less often. Many women who need emergency contraception are not good candidates for an IUD because they have yet to have children or currently have multiple partners and thus an elevated risk of PID.

Abortion

Q: Abortion isn't a form of contraception, but I'd like to know more about it anyway. What exactly is it?

A: Abortion is the termination of a pregnancy, and it can be done by various means. Most common in the United States is surgical abortion, the physical removal of the fetus from the uterus by a physician. The type of surgical abortion performed depends largely on how many weeks a woman has been carrying the fetus.

Medical abortion uses a combination of drugs to terminate pregnancy. First-trimester medical abortion has been available in Europe for a number of years and is now being performed in the United States at a few clinics.

Q: What types of surgical abortion are performed early in a pregnancy?

A: More than 90 percent of abortions in the United States are performed in the first trimester with a method called vacuum aspiration or suction curettage. The cervix is cleaned, anesthetized and dilated (widened), and a tube attached to a suction pump extracts the fetal tissue from the uterus. In some cases, a syringe can be used instead of a mechanical vacuum device. When necessary, an instrument called a curette is used to scrape the walls of the uterus to make sure it is empty. Done properly, this method of abortion is nearly 100 percent effective and rarely causes complications.

Q: What happens if a woman needs a second-trimester abortion?

A: Early second-trimester abortions require two steps. First, the cervix must be dilated. Then the uterus is evacuated. This method, known as dilation and evacuation (D&E), requires the insertion of special devices that cause the cervix to open up, a process that may take several hours. Some clinics may allow a woman to leave the clinic during this time. In either case, when the cervix is dilated, the woman returns to the clinic or hospital to have the contents of the uterus removed with a suction curette and other instruments. This part of the procedure takes 10 to 20 minutes and can be performed up to week 20 of pregnancy.

Q: What about late-term abortions—when and how are they performed?

A: Abortion after week 24 is quite rare, accounting for only one of every 10,000 cases, according to the Planned Parenthood Federation of America. Such abortions should be performed only when the mother is at risk or when there is a problem with the fetus. In the majority of late-term abortions, a doctor injects one of several solutions into the vagina or uterus to induce labor and cause a stillbirth. Alternately, some physicians employ a D&E method in which the cervix is dilated several times until the opening is wide enough to remove the fetus.

Q: What are the risks of surgical abortion?

A: Roughly one of every 200 women who have abortions suffers complications such as pelvic infection or incomplete abortion. Bleeding is common, but transfusion is required in less than one of every 500 cases. There is no evidence that suction curettage methods of abortion hinder a woman's ability to bear children in the future.

Abortion performed prior to eight weeks results in the death of the woman in only one of every 600,000 cases. This figure rises to one of every 17,000 for abortions performed between weeks 16 and 20, and one in 6,000 for abortions performed after week 21.

Q: How many surgical abortions are performed every year in the United States?

A: Almost half of all unwanted pregnancies end in an abortion, which translates to more than 1.3 million abortions per year. Thirty-one million legal abortions were performed between 1973 and 1994. At current rates, 43 percent of American women will have had an abortion by the age of 45. Fifty-five percent of all women who have abortions are 25 years old or younger.

Q: What is the procedure for medical abortion?

A: Medical abortion can be performed within the first six weeks of pregnancy with either of two drug combinations: methotrexate plus misoprostol or mifepristone plus misoprostol. The most well-known abortion drug, the French-made RU-486, contains mifepristone, which inhibits the hormones that allow a pregnancy to continue. Methotrexate (an anticancer drug) works by disrupting fetal cell division.

As of mid-1998, RU-486 was available in the United States only at 17 selected clinics. Methotrexate is approved by the FDA for the treatment of cancer, psoriasis and rheumatoid arthritis, but not for medical abortion. Nonetheless, several U.S. clinics use it for abortion.

Medical abortions are also performed in the second trimester using one of several agents such as misoprostol or saline solution.

INFERTILITY ISSUES

Fertility

Q: Now that we've talked about preventing pregnancy, let's talk about fertility. When does fertility begin?

A: A girl can become pregnant as soon as she begins ovulating (releasing eggs from her ovaries) and having menstrual periods. Most girls begin menstruating (**menarche**) between the ages of 12 and 14; however, the onset of menstruation varies widely and can be as early as age 10.

A boy's testicles begin to create sperm as he moves through puberty. This usually occurs between the ages of 11 and 17, but it may happen earlier. Once the production of sperm has begun, a boy has the potential to father a child.

Q: How long does fertility normally last?

A: As we mentioned earlier, a woman has all the eggs she will ever produce when she is born. The eggs mature in her ovaries, and each month during her fertile years one of those eggs is released. A woman loses her natural capacity to have children when she stops ovulating at menopause (menopause usually takes place between the ages of 45 and 55). Men, on the other hand, produce millions of new sperm each day throughout their lives, and millions are released with each ejaculation. A man can father children well into his 70s and 80s.

Q: What if a couple wants to conceive a child? What are the odds that a woman will become pregnant when no birth control method is used?

A: Among women who use no form of birth control, more than three-quarters will be pregnant within a year. As we stressed, the timing of intercourse in relation to ovulation is critical: The odds of conceiving a child with one act of unprotected intercourse range from zero at the start of the menstrual cycle to one in four on the day before ovulation. Researchers have also analyzed the odds based on frequency of intercourse. The percentage of couples achieving pregnancy in six months runs from 17 percent for a frequency of less than once a week to 51 percent for a frequency of three times a week.

Q: What can a couple do to increase the odds of conceiving a child?

A: The most important thing a couple can do to increase their odds of conceiving a child is to know when ovulation occurs and have vaginal intercourse in the days preceding and immediately after ovulation. Sexual position can also play a role in a couple's ability to conceive. For most women, the optimal position for conception is to lie on their backs with the pelvis slightly elevated. This allows semen to collect at the cervix. To further increase the probability of conception, a woman should remain lying down for 20 minutes after ejaculation.

Men can increase the amount of sperm in the ejaculate by abstaining from sexual activities—at least those that lead to ejaculation—for a period of several days before having sex. However, abstinence for periods of longer than a week may damage sperm.

Infertility

Q: When should a couple seek a medical opinion if they can't conceive?

A: Ability to conceive depends not as much on the frequency of intercourse as on its timing. If a couple has been aware of the woman's ovulation cycle and been sexually active around the time of ovulation, they should probably seek a medical opinion if they have not conceived within 12 months— or six months for those over age 35. The man will probably be evaluated first because the tests to determine his fertility status are cheaper, easier and less invasive than those required to fully diagnose an infertile woman.

Q: How are fertility problems diagnosed in men, and how are they treated?

A: An estimated 80 percent of all cases can be diagnosed by a combination of a physical exam, a medical history and an analysis of sperm. A medical history looks at such things as onset of puberty, past infection (mumps, for example) and current medications. The physical should include an examination of the size and texture of the testes in order to determine their ability to produce sperm properly.

If no problems are evident from the routine exam, it will be necessary to determine the number of viable sperm cells in the ejaculate. The single most common male fertility problem is **oligospermia**, or low sperm count. In rare cases, men will not be able to produce sperm at all.

Beyond estimating the number of sperm present in the ejaculate, a fertility specialist may also need to assess whether the sperm are formed normally and are capable of movement. To measure all of these factors, a man being evaluated for fertility issues generally will be asked to ejaculate into a specimen jar and deliver the sample to a lab within an hour or two. The sample is considered to be on the lower limit of the normal range if it has fewer than 20 million sperm per milliliter and if fewer than 50 percent of the sperm are alive, properly formed and capable of spontaneous movement.

Another method is to take a sample of cervical mucus from the woman immediately after the man has ejaculated into her vagina. This test is called a **postcoital test**. In addition to counting viable sperm, the postcoital test can determine whether the cervical mucus is receptive to sperm. Sometimes the mucus isn't the proper consistency and inhibits the movement of sperm in the reproductive tract.

Q: Let's go back a minute. What causes a low sperm count?

A: A number of factors affect the production of sperm. Sperm cells are very sensitive to heat and can be produced only at temperatures 3°F to 5°F cooler than the body (98.6°F). This is why the scrotum holds the testes outside and away from a man's body. In fact, some authorities say that wearing snugly fitting underwear that holds the testes too close to the body (and therefore raises their temperature) can lower sperm count.

Men may have difficulty producing sperm for a variety of other reasons. Previous infections such as mumps or diseases such as diabetes can hinder sperm production, as can hormone deficiencies. Various drugs and environmental factors can also decrease production. Lead poisoning and pesticide exposure are linked with low sperm count, for example, as are cigarette smoking, alcohol use and marijuana use. Certain prescription drugs may also damage sperm count or function.

Q: How are male fertility problems treated?

A: Compensating for male fertility problems generally depends on the number and viability of the sperm.

If sperm count is in the low end of the normal range, a couple may want to take extra measures. For example, they should be careful to time intercourse as closely as possible to ovulation. And the man should abstain from masturbation or lovemaking for three or four days prior to intercourse in order to allow his sperm count to rise.

If natural conception is not possible, a couple may want to try **artificial insemination.** In this technique, sperm is removed from the semen and introduced into the woman's reproductive tract through a special catheter during ovulation. If the man does not produce any sperm, the couple will need to rely on a sperm donor.

Q: What about women? What are the common causes of female infertility, and how are they diagnosed?

A: The most common causes of female infertility include lack of ovulation, blockage of the fallopian tubes and inability of the fertilized egg to implant in the wall of the uterus.

Lack of ovulation can be diagnosed through a blood test. Measuring progesterone levels in the blood is one of the most effective ways to determine if a woman is ovulating properly. Progesterone levels normally rise during ovulation.

Three techniques are generally used to check for blockage of the fallopian tubes and other physical damage to the reproductive system. The first, hysterosalpingography, is a procedure in which a physician injects a dye through the cervix and then follows the spread of the dye with an x-ray to see if it disperses throughout the reproductive organs. The second technique, laparoscopy, is a surgical procedure done under anesthesia that involves the insertion of a fiberoptic camera through the navel. The physician looks not only for blockage but also endometriosis and pelvic scarring. A third technique, transvaginal ultrasound, places a probe in the reproductive system and then follows its movements with ultrasound.

And to check if the uterine lining is suitable for implantation of a fertilized egg, a small sample of the uterine lining is taken (endometrial biopsy) on day 26 of the 28-day menstrual cycle. This is analyzed for the presence of sufficient progesterone to induce the necessary monthly uterine changes. Along with these exams, blood work is performed on the woman to check her hormone levels.

Q: How are these female fertility problems treated?

A: Problems with ovulation can usually be treated effectively with drug therapies. The two most common are clomiphene citrate, which reduces the ovulation-suppressive effect of estrogen, and bromocriptine, which helps keep the ovulation-suppressive effects of prolactin in check. Blockages in a woman's reproductive system often require surgical procedures, depending on the exact nature of the problem. Finally, progesterone will help make the uterus more receptive to implantation.

If these methods do not produce results, medical science has devised two other ways for causing pregnancy. A procedure called gamete intrafallopian tube transfer (GIFT) collects eggs and sperm and places them directly into the fallopian tube, where it is hoped fertilization will occur. It is used primarily for unexplained infertility, where the fallopian tubes appear to function normally.

In vitro fertilization (IVF) combines a sperm cell and an egg in a laboratory culture. Once the fertilized egg (called a zygote) has gone through six to eight cell divisions, it is transplanted into the woman's uterus. The overall live delivery rate per retrieval is 28 percent for GIFT versus 21 percent for IVF.

The final option for a couple unable to bear children is to engage a surrogate mother to carry the zygote, which has been started in vitro, and ultimately give birth to the child.

Q: We've covered a lot of territory. What else can you say about sexual health?

A: We have indeed covered a lot of ground. We have talked about the paradox of our society's obsession with sex combined with its avoidance of some of the most important health issues related to sexuality. We have described the key physiological processes of sexual response and sexual function—along with some of the medical problems that may prevent us from having or enjoying sex—and we have covered a variety of common sex-related infections and disorders. Last, we have described the physical process of conception and the ways that medical technology has offered us substantial control over how and when we create new life.

In ending on this last point, we are reminded that the anxieties, misconceptions and diseases that plague us today should not—and need not—be passed on to the next generation. When we see a young man or a young woman, we should consider that in a biological sense the next generation represents a clean slate, potentially disease-free. Without us, our children wouldn't be subject to AIDS or gonorrhea or syphilis—a sad legacy. Arguably, the same might be said for some of the psychosocial causes of sexual illness and dysfunction. What we hope we have argued persuasively here is that all of us have the opportunity to redefine our society's approach to sexual health. What's needed is a more open dialogue. We hope this book will give you the knowledge and help you find the words to make that happen.

APPENDIX

Internal Side View of the Male Reproductive System

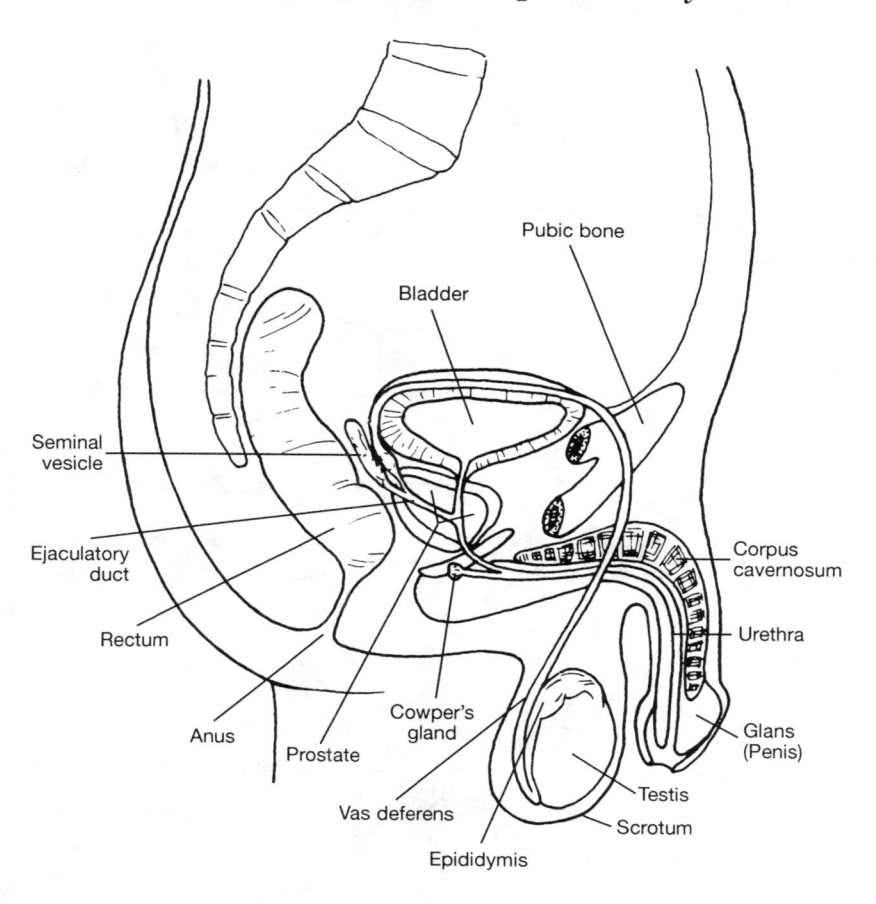

165

Internal Side View of the Female Reproductive System

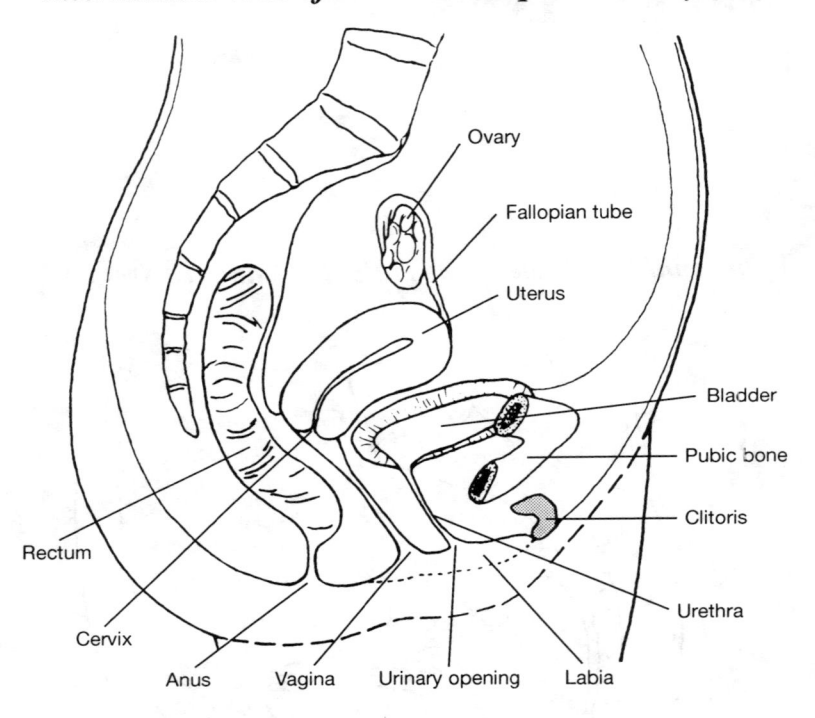

Exterior Reproductive Organs of the Female

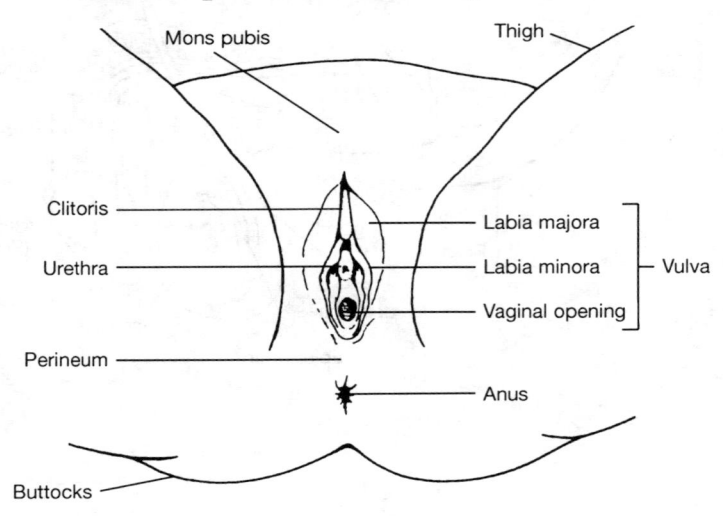

INFORMATIONAL AND MUTUAL-AID GROUPS

Advocates for Youth
1025 Vermont Ave., N.W., Suite 200
Washington, DC 20005
202-347-5700
http://www.advocatesforyouth.org

Alan Guttmacher Institute
120 Wall St.
New York, NY 10005
212-248-1111

American Association of Sex Educators, Counselors and Therapists
P.O. Box 328
Mount Vernon, IA 52314-0238

American Foundation for Urologic Disease
300 W. Pratt St., Suite 401
Baltimore, MD 21201
410-727-2908
800-828-7866
http://www.afud.org

American Social Health Association
P.O. Box 13827
Research Triangle Park, NC 27709-3827
800-230-6039
http://www.ashastd.org
Herpes Hotline
919-361-8448

Centers for Disease Control and Prevention
National STD Hotline
800-227-8922
National HIV/AIDS Hotline
800-342-2437 (English)
800-344-7432 (Spanish)
800-243-7889 (TTY)

Health Advice Company
2515 E. Highway 54
2200 Century Plaza, Suite 101
Durham, NC 27713
888-ADVICE-8
http://www.advicecenter.com

HIV/AIDS Treatment Information Service
P.O. Box 6303
Rockville, MD 20849-6303
800-HIV-0440
http://www.hivatis.org

Impotence World Association
10400 Little Patuxent Pkwy., Suite 485
Columbia, MD 21044
410-715-9605

National Women's Health Network
514 10th St., N.W., Suite 400
Washington, DC 20004
202-628-7814

Planned Parenthood Federation of America
810 Seventh Ave.
New York, NY 10019
800-230-PLAN
http://www.ppfa.org/ppfa

Resolve, Inc.
1310 Broadway
Somerville, MA 02144
617-623-0744

Sexual Information and Education Council of the United States (SIECUS)
130 W. 42nd St., Suite 2500
New York, NY 10036
212-819-9770
http://www.siecus.org

GLOSSARY

Abortion: The medical or surgical termination of a pregnancy.

Abstinence: The practice of refraining from sexual activity.

Acquired immune deficiency syndrome (AIDS): A condition that develops after the human immunodeficiency virus has sufficiently weakened the immune system. It is marked by a series of opportunistic infections and eventually ends in death. See also **Human immunodeficiency virus (HIV)**.

Anal intercourse: Intercourse in which the penis is inserted through the anus into the rectum of a partner.

Anorgasmia: The inability to reach orgasm.

Anticipatory anxiety: An emotional block to orgasm that occurs when a person wants an orgasm so much that it is difficult to relax, breathe normally and let it happen.

Anus: The opening of the rectum where solid waste leaves the body.

Aphrodisiac: A food, drink, drug, scent or device that claims to increase sexual desire or improve sexual performance.

Artificial insemination: A technique used to create pregnancy when natural conception is not possible. Sperm is removed from the semen and is placed, using a special catheter, into the woman's reproductive tract during ovulation.

Bacterial vaginosis (BV): A bacterial infection of the vagina caused by the decline in the population of healthy vaginal microbes and an upsurge in growth of anaerobic bacteria and other microbes. It is not usually accompanied by pain, redness or swelling of vaginal tissues but may cause abnormal odor or excessive discharge.

Bacteriuria: The presence of unusually large numbers of bacteria in the urine.

Bartholin's gland: One of two glands located on either side of the opening of the vagina that secretes a lubricating mucus.

Bisexuality: An attraction to both the same sex and the opposite sex.

Bladder: The hollow organ in the lower abdomen where urine is stored.

Cervical cap: A rigid rubber cap placed over the cervix as a means of contraception. The cap, when coupled with spermicide, acts as a barrier to sperm.

Cervix: The narrow opening of the uterus that leads to the vagina.

Chancre: A single, firm, round, usually painless sore appearing on the external genitalia, vagina, rectum, anus, mouth or lips as a symptom of syphilis.

Chlamydia: A bacterium responsible for a number of common infectious diseases, especially infections of the genital tract.

Circumcised: Describes a man whose foreskin, the flap of skin that covers the glans of the penis, has been removed.

Clitoris: The small, elongated, highly sensitive organ at the top of the vulva that is a source of sexual pleasure for women. The clitoris is similar to the penis in that it becomes engorged and erect during sexual stimulation.

Conception: The process in which sperm penetrates the female ovum and creates a zygote; the beginning of a pregnancy.

Condom: A sheath worn over the penis during intercourse to prevent pregnancy and the transmission of sexually transmitted disease.

Contraception: The prevention of conception or pregnancy.

Cowper's gland: One of two pea-size glands located near the prostate gland that produce a thick fluid.

Cross-dresser: One who dresses in the clothes of the opposite sex. Cross-dressing is predominantly done by males. See also **Transvestism**.

Cryptorchism: See **Undescended testis**.

Culture: A test used to diagnose many kinds of bacteria and viruses. A swab or sample of the microbe in question is placed in a special growth medium.

Cunnilingus: Oral stimulation of the female genitalia.

Cyst: A sac or capsule filled with fluid.

Cystitis: An infection of the bladder. See also **Urinary tract infection (UTI)**.

Depo-Provera: A hormonal contraceptive for women that is injected every 12 weeks to prevent pregnancy.

Diaphragm: A round, rubber dome that fits inside the vagina and covers the cervix as a means of contraception. The dome, when coupled with spermicide, acts as a barrier for sperm.

Digital rectal examination: A procedure in which a doctor inserts a lubricated, gloved finger into the rectum to check the prostate gland for hard or lumpy areas.

Dyspareunia: Painful intercourse arising from either psychological or physiological causes.

Dysuria: Painful urination.

Ejaculation: In men, a sudden discharge of semen during orgasm. Some women also report having ejaculations, which may consist of urine or a buildup of vaginal secretions.

Ejaculatory inevitability: The point during the cycle of sexual response at which a man is certain to have an orgasm and ejaculate.

Endometriosis: A condition marked by abnormal tissue growth outside the uterus.

Epididymis: The tightly coiled tubing inside the testes in which sperm mature.

Epididymitis: An acute form of testicular pain caused by inflammation of the epididymis. The condition is a major complication of chlamydia and gonorrhea and can result in sterility.

Erectile dysfunction (ED): In men, an inability to get an erection or sustain an erection through ejaculation.

Erection: The process through which the penis becomes rigid enough for penetrative intercourse.

Estrogen: The female sex hormone, produced chiefly by the ovaries in women and by the testes in men. Estrogen is responsible for the enlargement of the breasts, the widening of the hips and the development of other female characteristics at puberty, as well as the successful functioning of the female reproductive system.

Excitement: A term used by Masters and Johnson to describe the first phase of the sexual response cycle. Heart and breathing rates increase, skin becomes flushed and the nipples, penis, breasts and vulva become engorged or erect.

Fallopian tube: One of two tubelike structures through which eggs are channeled from the ovaries to the uterus.

Fellatio: Oral stimulation of the male genitalia.

Female condom: A cylinder of thin polyurethane that is inserted into the vagina and fits over the cervix as a means of contraception. The condom, also called a vaginal pouch, prevents sperm and sexually transmitted microbes from entering the vagina.

Fertility: The ability of a woman or couple to become pregnant and give birth.

Fertility awareness method: A method of contraception that relies on tracking the days immediately before and after ovulation and abstaining from sex during the period of possible conception. Specific methods include observing changes in body temperature and cervical mucus.

Fertilization: The union of an egg from the woman and a sperm from the man.

Fibroid tumor: A noncancerous tumor of fibrous and muscular tissue that occurs in the wall of the uterus.

Flora: The complex mix of microorganisms that are normally found in the vagina, the gut and the mouth.

Genital herpes: A sexually transmitted viral disease marked by outbreaks and periods of remission. The two types of herpes are herpes simplex type 1 and herpes simplex type 2. Type 1 typically causes painful mouth sores, while type 2 causes genital sores and itching, burning, tenderness and redness on the genitals. See also **Herpes simplex virus (HSV).**

GLOSSARY

Genital warts: See **Human papillomavirus (HPV)**.

Glans: The tip of the penis.

Gonorrhea: A sexually transmitted bacterial infection residing in mucous membranes and spread through unprotected intercourse. It often has no symptoms.

Grafenberg spot (G-spot): A dime-size area of highly sensitive tissue on the upper vaginal wall. It is considered by some to create arousal on par with clitoral stimulation.

Hematuria: The presence of blood in the urine.

Hepatitis: A viral infection that causes inflammation of the liver. The hepatitis B virus (HBV), the most prevalent form of the disease, is spread through contaminated blood, semen, vaginal secretions, stool and saliva.

Herpes simplex virus (HSV): A viral infection that can cause painful and recurrent ulcers in and around the mouth and genitals; spread through body-to-body contact. See also **Genital herpes**.

Heterosexuality: An attraction to the opposite sex.

HIV/AIDS: The term given to the closely related conditions human immunodeficiency virus (HIV) and acquired immune deficiency syndrome (AIDS). See also **Human immunodeficiency virus (HIV)** and **Acquired immune deficiency syndrome (AIDS)**.

Homosexuality: An attraction to the same sex.

Hormone: A substance produced by a gland that influences how the body works. Estrogen is the primary hormone that affects women's reproductive systems; testosterone is the primary hormone for men. See also **Estrogen** and **Testosterone**.

Hormone replacement therapy: The general term for the use of synthetic hormones to offset a particular hormone deficiency in a woman (usually using estrogen) or a man (usually using testosterone).

Human immunodeficiency virus (HIV): A sexually transmitted viral disease that attacks the immune system, triggering an onslaught of opportunistic infections known as acquired immune deficiency syndrome, or AIDS. See also **Acquired Immune Deficiency Syndrome (AIDS)**.

Human papillomavirus (HPV): The family of viruses that causes warts, including warts on the hands, feet and genital area. HPV is also implicated in genital tract cancers such as cervical cancer.

Hydrocele: An excess of fluid that collects in the scrotum between the testis and surrounding membranes and causes the scrotum to swell.

Incontinence: A person's inability to control urination.

Infertility: The inability to cause pregnancy or become pregnant and give birth after 12 consecutive months of effort to do so.

Intercourse: Sexual activity in which insertion of the penis is involved. The term usually refers to vaginal intercourse.

Intrauterine device (IUD): A small T-shaped contraceptive device that prevents fertilization. It may also be inserted after unprotected intercourse to prevent pregnancy. See also **Morning-after contraception.**

Kidney: One of two bean-shaped organs located on either side of the spinal column in the lower back. The kidneys filter waste products from blood and produce urine.

Labia majora: The large, fleshy lip of the vulva.

Labia minora: The small, fleshy lip of the vulva.

Libido: Sexual drive.

Loss of desire: A condition in which a person is unable to feel sexual desire. It is also called low desire, loss of libido and desire deficiency.

Lubrication: The wetness in the vagina that develops in response to sexual stimulation.

Masturbation: The self-stimulation of the genitals for sexual pleasure.

Menarche: The onset of a girl's first menstrual cycle.

Menopause: The natural and permanent cessation of menstruation. Menopause usually takes place between the ages of 45 and 55, although some women experience their last period in their 60s, and others in their 30s.

Menstruation: The part of the reproductive cycle of a woman during which the lining of the uterus exits the body as a flow of blood and tissue.

Morning-after contraception: Techniques used in case of an emergency to prevent the fertilized egg from implanting in the uterus. Two possible methods are an intrauterine device and morning-after pills. See also **Intrauterine device (IUD)** and **Morning-after pills**.

Morning-after pills: A series of pills containing high doses of synthetic estrogen that are taken after unprotected intercourse to prevent pregnancy. One dose is taken as soon as possible after intercourse, and a second dose follows after 12 hours.

Multiple orgasm: Two or more climaxes per single sex act.

Neurotransmitters: Hormonelike brain chemicals that conduct nerve signals among the brain cells.

Norplant: A hormonal contraceptive for women that is surgically implanted in the upper arm and provides protection against pregnancy for up to five years.

Oligospermia: Low sperm count; the most common fertility problem.

Oral contraceptive: A combination of synthetic estrogen and progestin that prevents ovulation and changes cervical mucus and the lining of a woman's uterus to prevent pregnancy.

Oral sex: Sexual activity involving the sex organs and the mouth.

Orchiectomy: The surgical removal of the testes.

Orchitis: An inflammation of the testes.

Orgasm: The culmination of sexual excitement characterized by strong feelings of pleasure and marked usually by ejaculation of semen by the male and by contractions in both the male and female.

Orgasmic platform: A marked swelling of the walls in the outer third of the vagina (near the vaginal opening) that occurs in women during the plateau phase of the sexual response cycle.

Ovary: One of a pair of female reproductive glands in which the eggs are formed and estrogen is produced. The ovaries are located in the lower abdomen on either side of the uterus.

Ovulation: The phase of the female menstrual cycle in which an ovary releases an egg. Ovulation occurs approximately two weeks prior to the onset of menstruation.

Ovum: The egg, or reproductive cell, of a woman.

Pap smear: A method of examining cells collected from the cervix for evidence of infection, inflammation, abnormal cells or cancer. It is also called a Pap test.

Pelvic inflammatory disease (PID): A gynecological condition caused by an infection (usually sexually transmitted) that spreads from the vagina to the upper reproductive tract in the pelvic cavity. PID can cause abscesses, constant pain in the genital tract, infertility and more frequent menstrual periods.

Penis: The reproductive and sex organ of a man. The spongy tissue of the penis fills with blood during sexual excitement, allowing the penis to become erect for intercourse and ejaculation. Urine also passes out of the body through the penis.

Perimenopause: The phase immediately before and after menopause.

Perineum: The area of skin between the genitals and the anus.

Peyronie's disease: A condition in which the spongy tissue within the penis weakens, causing the organ to bend to one side when erect.

Pheromone: A chemical secreted by various animals that affects behavior in other members of the species through scent. It is speculated that the human species produces pheromones that make men and women more attractive to one another.

Plateau: A term used by Masters and Johnson to describe the second phase of the sexual response cycle, a phase in which reaction to sexual stimulation intensifies.

Polyp: A mass of tissue that develops on the inside wall of a hollow organ.

Postcoital test: A test used to diagnose fertility problems in which a sample of cervical mucus is taken from a woman immediately after a man has ejaculated into her vagina. The test determines whether the sperm is viable and whether the mucus is receptive.

Premature ejaculation: In men, tendency to reach climax more quickly than is desired.

Priapism: A condition in which the penis remains erect for several hours, resulting in moderate pain and possibly permanent damage to the organ.

Progesterone: The female sex hormone associated with the thickening of the uterine lining.

Prostate cancer: A slow-growing cancer of the prostate gland.

Prostate gland: A doughnut-shaped gland that surrounds the urethra. The prostate produces a portion of the fluid that is found in semen.

Prostate-specific antigen (PSA): A substance—produced by prostate cells—whose level increases in the presence of prostate cancer.

Prostatitis: An inflammation of the prostate gland.

Pubic lice: Small parasites that can be sexually transmitted. Symptoms include intense itching of the genitals and anus.

Pyuria: The presence of pus in the urine.

Rectum: The portion of the large intestine between the colon and the anus.

Refractory period: The period of the sexual response cycle, lasting only a few minutes, during which a man is unable to have another climax even if the penis is still erect and stimulation continues.

Resolution: The last phase of the sexual response cycle as described by Masters and Johnson. Resolution immediately follows orgasm and consists of the time it takes for the body to return to its unaroused state.

Safer sex: The practice of preventing the transmission of sexually transmitted disease during sexual activity. It includes limiting activity to low-risk behaviors, as well as using male and female condoms for protection.

Scabies: An infection caused by the itch mite, a microscopic parasite that burrows into the skin and lays eggs. Scabies may be sexually transmitted.

Scrotum: The external sac of skin enclosing the testes.

Semen: The fluid produced in the testes that contains sperm, prostatic fluid and fluid from the seminal vesicles. Semen is released during sexual intercourse at ejaculation and is necessary for fertilization of the egg released by a woman at ovulation.

Seminal vesicle: A small sac connected to the urethra that produces a fluid that nourishes sperm and protects it from the acidity of vaginal secretions.

Sex: The reproductive act of vaginal intercourse; can also include other types of genital contact, such as oral or anal sex.

Sex flush: The pink or red blotches typically found around the breasts or elsewhere on the upper body during the excitement and plateau phases of the sexual response cycle. Sex flush occurs more often in women than in men.

Sexual health: The state that encompasses not only reproductive health also but the ability to appreciate one's own body, to interact with both genders in respectful ways and to express affection, love and intimacy in ways consistent with one's own values.

Sexual response cycle: The process through which the body goes during a sexual encounter. It consists of four stages: excitement, plateau, orgasm and resolution. See also **Excitement, Plateau, Orgasm** and **Resolution**.

Sexuality: The state created by a combination of sexual behaviors, desires and standards that affect one's emotional and physical life.

Sexually transmitted disease (STD): Any disease passed from person to person by sexual contact. Sexual contact includes all forms of penetrating intercourse, oral intercourse and a wide range of activities generally described as sex play.

Sperm: The male reproductive cell present in semen, released during ejaculation and capable of fertilizing the egg of the female. Sperm are produced in the testes.

Spermicide: A chemical foam, cream, film or jelly placed into the vagina and close to the cervix before intercourse as a means of contraception.

Sterilization: A nonreversible contraceptive method, usually involving surgery. See also **Tubal ligation** and **Vasectomy**.

Syphilis: A sexually transmitted infection that is still epidemic in some parts of the United States. Initial symptoms include sores called chancres and flulike symptoms. If left untreated, syphilis can result in heart disease, arthritis, brain damage, paralysis, blindness, dementia, impotency and even death.

Testes: The two egg-shaped glands situated in the scrotum that produce sperm and testosterone; also called testicles. A single gland is called a testis or testicle.

Testicular cancer: A rare form of cancer that affects the testes.

Testicular self-examination: A self-test in which a man gently feels the testes for any abnormal lumps or thickening that may indicate cancer.

Testicular torsion: The condition that occurs when one of the testes becomes twisted out of its normal position inside the scrotum. It can result in the kinking of blood vessels, which shuts down blood flow to and from the testis.

Testosterone: The most important male sex hormone. In men, it is produced in the testes and then released into the bloodstream. It is responsible for the development of the mature male body and initiates the production of sperm. After puberty, it helps to maintain sexual drive. In women, smaller amounts of testosterone are produced in the ovaries and are important to reproductive function.

Testosterone deficiency: The condition that occurs when the functioning of the testes is impaired or when there is a defect in the glands that stimulate testosterone production by the testes. Potential causes include aging, genetic abnormalities, infection or injury to the testes and certain medications.

Thrush: An overgrowth of yeast organisms in the throat and mouth.

Transsexual: One who views his or her gender as being the opposite of what anatomy would normally dictate. An example would be someone born with male genitals who feels he is instead a woman.

Transvestism: A specific type of cross-dressing in which (typically) a man dresses in women's clothing.

Trichomoniasis: A common infection caused by the microbe *Trichomonas vaginalis* that may be spread through sexual intercourse.

Tubal ligation: A method of permanent contraception for women that surgically closes off the fallopian tubes to prevent the egg from entering the uterus.

Uncircumcised: Describes a man whose foreskin, the flap of skin that covers the glans of the penis, is intact.

Undescended testis: In male infants, a condition in which one of the testes does not descend from the abdomen (where it has formed) into the scrotum. The condition can be surgically corrected but carries with it an increased risk of testicular cancer.

Urethra: The canal through which urine is discharged and, for the man, through which semen is discharged.

Urethritis: An inflammation of the urethra.

Urinary sphincter: The muscular opening of the bladder that controls the flow of urine out through the urethra.

Urinary tract: The organs and ducts involved in the elimination of urine from the body. It consists of the kidneys, ureters (the tubes connecting the kidneys and the bladder), bladder and urethra.

Urinary tract infection (UTI): An infection of the urinary tract. See also **Cystitis** and **Urethritis**.

Uterus: In women, the hollow, muscular organ located in the pelvic cavity in which the fertilized egg implants and develops. It is also referred to as the womb.

Vagina: In women, the flexible, muscular passage that leads from the uterus to the outside of the body. It is through the vagina that the menstrual flow passes and through which a fetus is born. It also receives the penis during vaginal intercourse.

Vaginismus: An involuntary, painful and usually prolonged contraction of the vagina. Its causes can be psychological or physiological.

Vaginitis: An inflammation of the vaginal tissue accompanied by itching, discharge, a fishy odor and other symptoms. It may or may not be related to sexually transmitted organisms.

Vas deferens: In men, the two tubelike structures that each connect a testicle to the urethra. The interior end of the vas deferens serves as a duct in which sperm can collect before ejaculation.

Vasectomy: A method of permanent contraception for men that involves surgically cutting the vas deferens to prevent sperm from mixing with the semen.

Vasocongestion: An increased flow of blood in a part of the body (for example, the penis).

Venereal disease: See **Sexually transmitted disease (STD)**.

Vesicle: A clear, dome-shaped blister often associated with oral or genital herpes.

Vibrator: An electronic, vibrating device used to stimulate either external or internal genitalia of a man or woman.

Vulva: The exterior genitalia of a woman.

Vulvar pruritits: An itching of the vulva.

Vulvovaginal candidiasis (VVC): A fungal infection of the vagina and vulva caused by *Candida albicans* or other yeasts; often called a yeast infection.

Withdrawal: The withdrawal of the penis before ejaculation. It is a highly unreliable contraceptive method.

Yeast infection: A fungal infection caused by *Candida albicans* or other yeasts. Symptoms of oral and vaginal infections include pain, itching, redness and white patches in their respective sites. See also **Vulvovaginal candidiasis (VVC)**.

Yohimbine: An African tree-bark extract that can produce warm spinal shivers and pelvic tingles. It is primarily used to treat male erectile dysfunction because of its ability to open up penile blood vessels.

SUGGESTED READING

Barbach, Lonnie. *For Each Other.* New York: Anchor, 1982.

Ebel, Charles. *Managing Herpes: How to Live and Love With a Chronic STD.* Research Triangle Park, N.C.: American Social Health Association, 1994.

Eng, Thomas R., and William T. Butler. *The Hidden Epidemic: Confronting Sexually Transmitted Diseases.* Washington, D.C.: National Academy Press, 1997.

Guillebaud, John. *Contraception: Your Questions Answered.* New York: Churchill Livingstone, 1993.

Hatcher, Robert A., et al. *Contraceptive Technology.* New York: Ardent Media, 1998.

Heiman, Julia R., and Joseph Lopiccolo. *Becoming Orgasmic: A Sexual and Personal Growth Program for Women.* New York: Fireside, 1976.

Holmes, King K., et al. *Sexually Transmitted Diseases.* New York: McGraw-Hill, 1990.

Love, Susan M., and Karen Lindsey. *Dr. Susan Love's Hormone Book.* New York: Random House, 1998.

Michael, Robert T., et al. *Sex in America: A Definitive Survey.* New York: Warner, 1994.

Nachtigall, Lila E., and Joan Rattner Heilman. *Estrogen: The Facts Can Change Your Life.* New York: Harper Perennial, 1995.

Reinisch, June M., and Ruth Beasley. *The Kinsey Insititute New Report on Sex.* New York: St. Martin's, 1990.

Schwartz, Pepper, and Virginia Rutter. *The Gender of Sexuality.* Thousand Oaks, Calif.: Pine Forge, 1998.

Zilbergeld, Bernie. *The New Male Sexuality.* New York: Bantam, 1992.

INDEX

A

Abortion
  defined, 11, 155, 169
  early, 155-156
  incidence, 156-157
  late-term, 156
  medical, 157
  risks with surgical, 156-157
  second-trimester, 156
Abstinence, defined, 13, 169
Acquired immune deficiency syndrome.
  See AIDS
Acyclovir, effects, 85, 86
Adolescents. *See* Teenagers
Aging
  effects on erections, 59-60
  effects on orgasm, 40, 49
  men and sexuality, 49, 59-62
  sexual activity, 13-14, 25, 49
  women and sexuality, 44-49
AIDS
  defined, 67, 95, 169
  long-term risks, 69
  media role in education, 20
  transmission, 99
  treatment, 99
  vs. HIV, 95, 98
Alcohol, effects, 52, 65
Alcoholism, effects, 53
Aldactone, effects, 54
Aldara, effects, 90
Aldomet, effects, 54
Alprostadil, effects, 57
Alzheimer's disease, hormone replacement
  therapy effects, 47
Amphetamine, effects, 64
Anafranil, effects, 54
Anal cancer, causes, 92
Anal intercourse
  defined, 25, 169
  prevalence, 25
  risks, 92, 104, 130
Anorgasmia
  causes, 39, 40-41, 49-50
  defined, 39, 169
  men, 49-52
  treatment, 40-41, 50-51

Antibiotics
  bacterial vaginosis, 113-114
  chlamydia, 71-72, 74-75
  epididymitis, 130
  gonorrhea, 74-75
  pelvic inflammatory disease, 76
  prostatitis, 127
  syphilis, 76, 77
  trichomoniasis, 79
  urinary tract infection, 124
  yeast infection, 117
Anticipatory anxiety, defined, 40, 169
Antidepressants
  effects, 43-44, 54, 63
  side effects, 50
Antifungal agents, effects, 119-120
Antihistamines, effects, 43-44, 80
Antihypertensives, effects, 54
Antipsychotics, effects, 54
Antiviral therapy, suppressive, effects,
  86, 87, 89
Anus, defined, 27, 169
Anxiety, effects, 49, 52, 65
Aphrodisiacs
  defined, 64, 169
  effects, 64-65
Aqualube, effects, 44, 48
Arousal, sexual
  physical changes
    men, 31-35
    women, 35-37
  triggers, 31
Arthritis, causes, 77
Artificial insemination, defined, 161, 169
Astroglide, effects, 44, 48
Azithromycin, effects with chlamydia, 71-72
AZT, effects, 98

B

Bacterial vaginosis
  causes, 109-112
  defined, 78, 109-110, 169
  diagnosis, 112-113
  long-term effects, 114
  prevalence, 112
  prevention, 115-116
  risk factors, 111
  symptoms, 112-113, 115-116

183

treatment, 113-116
  male partners, 115
  vs. yeast infection, 116
Bacteriuria, defined, 122, 169
Bartholin's glands, defined, 35, 170
Basal body temperature method, defined, 152
Bendroflumethiazide, effects, 54
Bichloracetic acid, effects, 90
Biochemical research, pheromones, 65, 176
Biopsy, prostate cancer, 128
Birth control pill
  effects, 43-44, 142
  men, 146
  pros/cons, 142-143
Bisexuality
  defined, 21, 170
  determination, 22
Bladder, defined, 32, 170
Bladder problems, effects, 53
Blindness, causes, 77
Blood pressure, high, effects, 53, 63
Brain damage, causes, 77
Breast cancer
  causes, 142
  hormone replacement therapy, 47-48
Breastfeeding, effects, 43-44, 154
Bromocriptine, effects, 162
Butoconazole, effects, 119-120
BV. See Bacterial vaginosis

C
Calendar method. See Rhythm method
Cancer
  anal, causes, 92
  breast, causes, 47-48, 142
  cervical
    causes, 91
    STD role, 69
  chemotherapy, effects, 61, 63
  colon, causes, 47
  endometrial, causes, 142
  ovarian, causes, 142
  penile, causes, 92
  prostate
    death rates, 128
    defined, 109, 177
    diagnosis, 128
    incidence, 128
    risk factors, 128
    symptoms, 128
    treatment, 128-129
  testicular
    defined, 109, 179
    incidence, 132
    risk factors, 132
    survival rates, 132-133
    symptoms, 133
    treatment, 133
Catapres, effects, 54

Catheterization, prostatitis, 127
Cervical cancer
  causes, 91
  STD role, 69
Cervical cap
  defined, 140, 170
  pros/cons, 151
  vs. diaphragm, 151
Cervix, defined, 17, 170
Chancre, defined, 76, 170
Chemotherapy
  effects, 61, 63
  prostate cancer, 129
  testicular cancer, 133
Children, urinary tract infection, 122
Chlamydia
  causes, 67
  defined, 43, 170
  diagnosis, 71
  effects, 130
  fertility, 71, 72, 105
  long-term effects, 70-71
  during pregnancy, 106
  prevalence, 69, 70
  symptoms, 71, 74-75, 75, 123
  treatment, 71-72, 74-75
Chlorine, effects, 118
Chlorothiazide, effects, 54
Chocolate, effects, 64
Chronic illness, effects on sexual function, 14
Circumcised, defined, 118, 170
Cleocin, effects, 113
Clindamycin, effects, 113
Clitoris
  defined, 35, 170
  role in sexual function, 36, 37
  stimulation, techniques, 39
Clomiphene citrate, effects, 162
Clomipramine, effects, 54
Clonidine, effects, 54
Clothing, tight, effects, 117, 121
Clotrimazole, effects, 119-120
Coffee, effects, 87-88
Cold medications, OTC, side effects, 43-44
Colon cancer, causes, 47
Computed tomography (CT), prostate cancer, 128
Conception, defined, 137, 170
Condom
  breakage/slippage, 148
  defined, 12, 146, 170
  effectiveness for contraceptive use, 147
  female
    contraception, 149-150
    defined, 149, 172
    pros/cons, 149-150
    STD protection, 100
  guidelines for contraceptive use, 146
  herpes, 87

pros/cons, 147
STD prevention, 93, 100-102, 115
STDs during pregnancy, 106
types, 100-101, 146, 148-149
urinary tract infection, 123-124
use guidelines, 101-102
Condylox, effects, 90
Contraception. *See also* Tubal ligation;
Vasectomy
alcohol effects, 65
barrier methods. *See* Cervical cap;
Condom; Diaphragm; IUD;
Spermicide
burden on women, 17
defined, 27, 140, 170
drug abuse effects, 65
emergency, 154-155
hormonal methods. *See* Birth control pill;
Implants; Injectables
making choices, 140-141
perfect vs. typical use, 141
Corticosteroids, effects, 120, 131
Cowper's glands, defined, 34, 170
Crabs. *See* Pubic lice
Crixivan, effects, 99
Cross-dresser, defined, 23, 170
Cryotherapy, effects, 90
Cryptorchism, defined. *See* Undescended testis
Culture, defined, 171
Cunnilingus, defined, 39, 171
Cystitis
defined, 122, 171
honeymoon, 123
Cysts, defined, 44, 171

D

ddC, effects, 98
ddI, effects, 98
Delavirdine, effects, 99
Dementia, causes, 77
Dental dam, defined, 103
Depo-Provera, defined, 144-145, 171
Depression, effects, 14, 54, 63
Diabetes, effects, 14, 53, 117, 120, 142
Diaphragm
defined, 27, 150, 171
pros/cons, 150-151
vs. female condom, 150
Diflucan, effects, 119-120
Digital rectal exam (DRE)
American Cancer Society recommendations, 129
defined, 128, 171
Diupres, effects, 54
Diuretics, effects, 54
Diuril, effects, 54
Doryx, effects, 71-72
Douching, effects, 75, 110, 118, 121
Doxycycline hydrochloride, effects with chlamydia, 71-72

Drug abuse, effects, 50, 53, 65
Dryness, vaginal
causes, 43-44
incidence, 46
Dyspareunia
causes, 43-44
defined, 43, 171
incidence, 46
Dysuria, defined, 118, 171

E

Eating disorders, prevalence, 20
ED. *See* Erectile dysfunction
Education
AIDS, media role, 20
effect on STD prevalence, 11-12
effect on unintended pregnancy incidence, 13
school-based sexual, 19
sexual orientation, media role, 20
Ejaculation
defined, 14, 171
premature
defined, 49, 51, 177
treatment, 51-52
sequence of events, 34
women, 37
Ejaculatory inevitability. *See also* Orgasm
defined, 33, 171
Elimite, effects, 80
Emergency contraception, 154-155
Empowerment, sexual health, 29
Endometrial cancer, causes, 142
Endometriosis, defined, 44, 171
Epididymis, defined, 33, 171
Epididymitis
causes/treatment, 130
defined, 109, 130, 171
long-term effects, 130
symptoms, 130
Epilepsy, effects, 63
Erectile dysfunction
aging, 59-60
causes, 53-55, 129
defined, 52, 171
diagnostic tests, 55
incidence, 53
treatment, 55-60
Erectile problems, men, 52-60
Erection
defined, 32, 171
medical aid, 14
Eskalith, effects, 54
Estrogen. *See also* Hormone replacement therapy
birth control pill, 141
defined, 44, 172
effects, 117, 121
forms, 46-47
role in female reproductive system, 44-45
role in sexual arousal, 45

Excitement
 defined, 32, 172
 physical changes
  men, 32
  women, 35-38

F

Fallopian tube blockage, effects, 70, 76, 161
Fallopian tubes, defined, 45, 172
Famciclovir, effects, 85
Famvir, effects, 85
Fatigue, effects, 52, 65
Fellatio, defined, 100, 172
Feminine hygiene sprays, effects, 118
Femstat, effects, 119-120
Fertility. *See also* Infertility
 after contraception, 145
 chlamydia, 71, 72, 105
 conception odds, 158-159
 defined, 24, 172
 peak age, 24, 157-158
Fertility awareness method
 defined, 152, 172
 effectiveness, 153-154
Fertilization, defined, 137-138, 172
Fibroid tumor, defined, 44, 172
Flagyl, effects, 79, 113
Flora, defined, 110, 172
Fluconazole, effects, 119-120
Fluoxetine, side effects, 50
Fluphenazine, effects, 54
Fluvoxamine, side effects, 50
Folic acid deficiencies, effects, 93

G

G-spot, defined, 40, 173
Gamete intrafallopian tube transfer (GIFT),
 defined, 162
Genital herpes. *See* Herpes, genital
Genital warts. *See* Warts, genital
Glans, defined, 52, 173
Gonorrhea
 causes, 67, 114
 defined, 43, 173
 diagnosis, 74
 effects, 130
 long-term effects, 73
 during pregnancy, 106
 prevalence, 72-73
 symptoms, 73, 74-75, 123
 transmission, 73, 102
 treatment, 74-75
Grafenberg spot. *See* G-spot
Guanethidine, effects, 54

H

Hardening of the arteries, effects, 53
Health care services access
 effect on STD prevalence, 11-12
 effect on unintended pregnancy
  incidence, 13

Heart disease
 causes, 77
 effects, 53
 hormone replacement therapy effects,
  47, 48
Hepatitis
 defined, 93, 173
 symptoms/diagnosis/treatment, 94
 transmission, 93-94
 vaccine, 94-95
Herpes
 causes, 67
 genital
  causes, 88, 89
  defined, 11, 172
  diagnosis, 84-85
  HIV-related, 96
  during pregnancy, 106
  prevalence, 81
  primary episode, 82
  symptoms, 82-83, 87-88, 123
  transmission, 86-87, 102, 103, 105
  treatment, 85-86
 herpes simplex virus
  defined, 81, 173
  types, 84-85
 prevalence, 70
Herpes simplex virus
 defined, 81, 173
 types, 84-85
Heterosexuality, defined, 21, 173
HIV
 causes, 67, 114
 defined, 67, 95, 173
 diagnosis, 96, 97-98
 long-term risks, 69
 opportunistic infections, 96
 during pregnancy, 106
 symptoms, 96
 transmission, 95-96, 99
 vs. AIDS, 95, 98
Hivid, effects, 98
Homosexuality, defined, 21, 173
Honeymoon cystitis/bladder, 123
Hormonal problems, effects, 53
Hormone deficiency, men, 53, 60-63
Hormone replacement therapy. *See also*
  Estrogen; Progesterone
 defined, 46, 173
 pros/cons, 47-48
Hormones, defined, 25, 173
Hot flash, incidence, 45
Hot tubs, effects, 68
HPV
 cervical, treatment, 92-93
 defined, 174
 diagnosis, 92
 prevalence, 70
 prevention, 93
 transmission, 103, 105
HRT. *See* Hormone replacement therapy

INDEX 187

HSV. *See* Herpes simplex virus
Human immunodeficiency virus. *See* HIV
Human papillomavirus. *See* HPV
Hydrocele
 defined, 135, 174
 treatment, 135
Hysterosalpingography, infertilty, 161

I

Imiquimod, effects, 90
Immunosuppressive agents, effects, 120
Implants
 effectiveness, 141, 145
 penile, pros/cons, 58-59
 pros/cons, 145-146
Impotence. *See also* Erectile
  dysfunction (ED)
 causes, 77, 129
 defined, 52
In vitro fertilization (IVF), defined, 162
Incontinence, urinary
 causes, 129
 defined, 129, 174
Inderal, effects, 54
Indinavir, effects, 99
Infections, dyspareunia, 43
Infertility. *See also* Fertility
 causes, 70, 76
 defined, 70, 174
 epididymitis, 130
 female, 161-162
 medical attention, 159
 men, 159-161
 orchitis, 131
Informational and mutual-aid groups,
  contact information, 167-168
Injectables. *See also* Depo-Provera;
  Norplant
 effectiveness, 145
 men, 146
 pros/cons, 145-146
Injection, penile
 costs, 58
 effects, 56, 57-58
Intercourse. *See also* Anal intercourse;
  Sexual intercourse; Vaginal
  intercourse
 defined, 14, 174
 painful. *See* Dyspareunia
Interferon, effects, 94
Intrauterine device. *See* IUD
Invirase, effects, 99
Isemelin, effects, 54
IUD
 defined, 111, 143, 174
 effectiveness, 144
 emergency contraception, 154, 155
 pros/cons, 144
 risks, 111
 safety issues, 143

K

K-Y Jelly, effects, 44, 48
Kidney, defined, 122, 174
Kidney problems, effects, 53
Kildane, effects, 80
Kinsey, Alfred, sexuality research, 21
Kissing, herpes simplex type 1, 88

L

Labia majora, defined, 35, 174
Labia minora, defined, 35, 174
Lactobacillus-containing capsules,
  effects, 114
Levonorgestrel. *See* Norplant
Libido. *See also* Loss of desire; Sexual drive
 defined, 63, 174
Lice, pubic. *See* Pubic lice
Lindane, effects, 80
Lithium, effects, 54
Liver disease, STD role, 69
Loop electrosurgical excision procedure
  (LEEP), cervical HPV, 92-93
Loss of desire. *See also* Libido; Sexual drive
 defined, 49, 63, 174
Lotrimin, effects, 119-120
Lubrication
 defined, 35, 174
 inadequate, 43-44
Luvox, side effects, 50
Lysine, effects, 88-89

M

Magnetic resonance imaging (MRI),
  prostate cancer, 128
Married couples, sexual intercourse
  frequency, 24
Masturbation
 defined, 10, 174
 effects, 26
 orgasm, 41, 51
 premature ejaculation, 51-52
 prevalence, 26
 prostatitis, 126
Media, effects on sexual health, 19-20
Medical establishment, role in sexual
  health, 16-17
Medications, effects, 54
Medroxyprogesterone acetate suspension.
  See Depo-Provera
Mellaril, effects, 54
Memory function, hormone replacement
  therapy effects, 47
Men
 aging and sexuality, 49, 59-62
 anorgasmia, 49-52
 contraceptives
  birth control pill, 146
  condom, 146-149
  injectables, 146
 erectile problems, 52-60

excitement, physical changes, 32
hormone deficiency, 53, 60-63
infertility, 159-161
orgasm, 33-35, 37-38
plateau effects, 33-34
problems of desire, 63-65
reproductive system, anatomical
  illustration, 165
reproductive tract disorders. *See*
  Epididymitis; Hydrocele; Orchitis;
  Peyronie's disease; Prostate cancer;
  Prostatitis; Testicular cancer;
  Testicular torsion
role in sexual health, 17
sexual arousal, physical changes, 31-35
urinary tract infection 124-125
yeast infections, 118-119
Menarche, defined, 158, 174
Menopause
  age range, 45
  causes, 45
  defined, 13, 174
  effects on sexual function, 13
  hormone replacement therapy, 46-49
  impacts on sexuality, 45-46
  peri-, defined, 45, 176
  symptoms, 45
  therapy, 46, 49
Menstrual cycle, average, 138
Menstruation
  causes, 139
  defined, 44, 175
Methotrexate, abortion, 157
Methyldopa, effects, 54
Metizol, effects, 79, 113
Metronidazole, effects, 79, 113-114
Miconazole, effects, 119-120
Misoprostol, abortion, 157
Monistat, effects, 119-120
Monodox, effects with chlamydia, 71-72
Mood-altering drugs, side effects, 50
Morning-after contraception, defined,
  154, 175
Morning-after pills, defined, 154, 175
Mucus method, defined, 152-153
Multiple orgasm
  defined, 37, 175
  drawbacks, 42
  incidence, 37
  techniques, 42
Mumps, effects, 131
Muscle relaxants, effects, 127
Muse, effects, 57
Mycelex, effects, 119-120
Mycostatin, effects, 119-120

N

Nardil, effects, 54
Naturetin, effects, 54
Nelfinavir, effects, 99

Nerve injuries, effects, 53
Neurotransmitters, defined, 31, 175
Nevirapine, effects, 99
Nilstat, effects, 119-120
Nipples, effects in plateau phase, 36
Nix, effects, 80
Nocturnal penile tumescence (NPT),
  defined, 55
Norplant, defined, 144, 145, 175
Norvir, effects, 99
Nucleoside reverse transcriptase (RT)
  inhibitors, effects, 98
Nutritional deficiencies, effects, 93
Nystatin, effects, 119-120

O

Obesity, effects, 142
Oligospermia, defined, 159, 175
Oral contraceptives. *See also* Birth
  control pill
  defined, 141, 175
Oral sex. *See also* Cunnilingus; Fellatio
  clitoral stimulation, 39
  condom, 100, 103
  defined, 25, 175
  genital herpes, 88
  incidence, 25
  risk levels, 104
  STDs, 72, 73, 100, 102-103
Orchiectomy, defined, 133, 175
Orchitis
  causes, 131
  defined, 109, 131, 175
  symptoms/treatment, 131
Orgasm. *See also* Anorgasmia; Ejaculatory
    inevitability
  age effects, 40, 49
  defined, 9, 173
  incidence, 38
  men, 33-35, 37-38
  multiple
    defined, 37, 175
    drawbacks, 42
    incidence, 37
    techniques, 42
  techniques, 39-43
  women, 13, 14, 37-43
Orgasmic platform, defined, 36, 175
Osteoporosis, hormone replacement
  therapy effects, 47, 48
Outercourse, defined, 103
Ovarian cancer, causes, 142
Ovary, defined, 45, 175
Ovulation
  defined, 24, 138, 176
  lack of, effects, 161
  schedule, 138
Ovum, defined, 137, 176

P

Painful intercourse. *See* Dyspareunia
Pap smears
  defined, 17, 176
  genital warts, 91-92
Papaverine, effects, 55
Paralysis, causes, 77
Parasites. *See* Pubic lice; Scabies
Parenting
  effects on sexual function, 13
  role in sexual health, 18-19
Paroxetine, side effects, 50
Paxil, side effects, 50
PEA. *See* Phenylethylamine
Pelvic inflammatory disease
  causes, 75
  defined, 43, 176
  IUD, 144
  symptoms/treatment, 75
Penicillin, effects, 76, 77
Penile cancer, causes, 92
Penile implants, pros/cons, 58-59
Penile injection
  costs, 58
  effects, 56, 57-58
Penis, defined, 31, 176
Perimenopause, defined, 45, 176
Perineum, defined, 126, 176
Permethrin, effects, 80
Peyronie's disease
  causes/treatment, 130
  defined, 125, 129, 176
Phenelzine, effects, 54
Phenylethylamine, effects, 64
Pheromones, defined, 65, 176
Physicians, role in sexual health, 16-17
PID. *See* Pelvic inflammatory disease
Plateau
  defined, 32, 176
  effects in men, 33-34
  physical changes, women, 36
Pneumonia, HIV-related, 96
Podofilox, effects, 90
Polyps, defined, 44, 176
Postcoital test, defined, 160, 176
Pregnancy
  bacterial vaginosis, 114, 115
  ectopic
    bacterial vaginosis, 114
    causes, 70-71
    defined, 70-71
  effects, 13, 117
  STDs during, 106
  unintended, incidence, 11, 13
  yeast infection, 121
Premature ejaculation
  defined, 49, 51, 177
  treatment, 51-52
Priapism
  defined, 56-57, 177
  penile injection, 58
  Viagra, 56-57
Progesterone. *See also* Hormone replacement therapy
  birth control pill, 141
  defined, 45, 177
  effects on infertility, 161
  forms, 47
Prolixin, effects, 54
Propranolol, effects, 54
Prostaglandin, effects, 55, 57
Prostat, effects, 113
Prostate cancer
  American Cancer Society recommendations, 129
  death rates, 128
  defined, 109, 177
  diagnosis, 128
  incidence, 128
  risk factors, 128
  symptoms, 128
  treatment, 128-129
Prostate gland, defined, 34, 177
Prostate-specific antigen (PSA)
  American Cancer Society recommendations, 129
  defined, 128, 177
Prostatectomy
  defined, 128-129
  prostate cancer, 128-129
Prostatitis
  acute bacterial, 125, 127
  causes, 125-126
  chronic bacterial, 125, 127
  congestive, 125-127
  defined, 109, 125, 177
  nonbacterial, 125-127
  prevalence, 125-127
  prostatodynia, 125-127
  symptoms, 126, 127
  treatment, 126-127
  types, 125
Prostheses, effects, 56
Protease inhibitors, effects, 99
Protostat, effects on trichomoniasis, 79
Prozac, side effects, 50
Psychotherapy, effects, 127
Pubic lice
  defined, 79, 177
  diagnosis/treatment, 80
  symptoms, 79
Pyuria, defined, 122, 177

R

Radiation therapy
  effects, 61
  prostate cancer, 129
  testicular cancer, 133
Recreational sex, defined, 9
Rectum, defined, 76, 177

Refractory period, defined, 38, 177
Relationship problems, effects, 64
Reproductive system
  female, anatomical illustration, 166
  male, anatomical illustration, 165
Reproductive tract disorders. *See* Bacterial vaginosis; Urinary tract infection; Yeast infection
STD role, 69
Rescriptor, effects, 99
Reserpine, effects, 54
Resolution, defined, 32, 177
Retrovir, effects, 98
Rhythm method, defined, 152
Ritonavir, effects, 99
RT inhibitors, effects, 98
RU-486, abortion, 157

S

Safer sex
  alcohol effects, 65
  defined, 27, 177
  drug abuse effects, 65
  guidelines, 100-101
  prospective partners, 107-108
  sexual activities, risk levels, 104
Saline solution, abortion, 157
Saquinivir, effects, 99
Scabene, effects, 80
Scabies
  defined, 79, 177
  diagnosis/treatment, 80
  symptoms, 79
School-based sexual education, 19
Scrotum, defined, 33, 177
Selective serotonin reuptake inhibitors (SSRIs), side effects, 50
Semen
  defined, 34, 178
  role in conception, 139
Seminal vesicles, defined, 34, 178
Sertraline, side effects, 50
Sex
  defined, 9, 178
  recreational, defined, 9
Sex flush
  defined, 33, 178
  women, 36
Sex toys, prevalence of use, 27
Sexual activity
  average age, 14-15
  risk levels, 104
Sexual arousal
  physical changes
    men, 31-35
    women, 35-37
  role of estrogen, 45
  triggers, 31
Sexual drive
  decreased, 45
  loss of desire, 49, 63, 174

peak age, 23
Sexual education, school-based, 19
Sexual function, problems, 13-14
Sexual health
  defined, 10, 178
  effects, 28
  empowerment, 29
Sexual identity, defined, 21
Sexual intercourse. *See also* Anal intercourse; Safer sex; Vaginal intercourse
  frequency, 24
  prostatitis, 126
  risk levels, 104
Sexual orientation
  defined, 21
  determination, 22
  media role in education, 20
Sexual relationships
  delayed ejaculation effects, 50
  prospective partners and safer sex, 107-108
Sexual response cycle. *See also* Excitement; Orgasm; Plateau; Resolution
  defined, 31, 178
Sexual revolution, effects, 14
Sexuality
  defined, 10, 178
  medical establishment role, 16-17
Sexually transmitted disease. *See* STD
Sildenafil. *See* Viagra
Single people, sexual intercourse frequency, 24
Smoking, effects, 53, 93, 142
Society, sexual health, 10-16
Sperm
  defined, 24, 178
  life span, 139
Sperm count, low, causes, 160
Spermicide
  defined, 27, 102, 178
  effects, 102, 118, 121
Spinal cord injuries, effects, 53
Spirinolactone, effects, 54
STD. *See also* AIDS; Bacterial vaginosis; Chlamydia; Gonorrhea; Hepatitis; Herpes; HIV; HPV; Pelvic inflammatory disease; Pubic lice; Scabies; Syphilis; Trichomoniasis; Vaginitis; Yeast infection
  avoidance guidelines, 100-101
  burden on women, 17-18
  causes of high prevalence, 12, 68
  common, 67, 69
  defined, 11, 67, 178
  effects, 43
  IUD, 144
  long-term risks, 69
  oral sex, 72, 73
  during pregnancy, 106
  prevalence, 11-12, 68, 105
  prevention, 27-28
  prospective partners, 107-108

INDEX

screening, 105
sexual activities, risk levels, 104
sexual activity with, 105
symptoms, 68-69
transmission, 67-68
Sterilization, defined, 140, 178
Stress, effects, 54
Stroke, birth control pill, 142
Suppositories
 urethral
  costs, 57
  effects, 56, 57
 vaginal, effects, 119-120
Surgery
 loop electrosurgical excision procedure (LEEP), cervical HPV, 92-93
 testicular cancer, 133
 testicular torsion, 135
 tubal ligation, 140, 180
 vascular, effects, 56
 vasectomy, 140, 181
Surrogate mothers, infertility options, 162
Swimming pools, effects, 118
Symptothermal method, defined, 153
Syphilis
 defined, 69, 179
 diagnosis, 77
 history, 76
 long-term effects, 77
 during pregnancy, 106
 prevalence, 76
 symptoms, 76-77
 transmission, 76
 treatment, 76, 77

T

Tampons, side effects, 43-44
Teenagers
 attitudes on sexuality, 19-20, 40
 double standard, 15-16
 eating disorders, 20
 girls, attitudes on sexuality, 19-20, 40
 knowledge sources, 19
 sexual activity, 14-16
 sexually active, urinary tract infection, 122
 STD, 12
 unintended pregnancy, 11, 13
Testes
 defined, 32, 179
 role in sexual function, 32
Testicular cancer
 defined, 109, 179
 incidence, 132
 risk factors, 132
 survival rates, 132-133
 symptoms/treatment, 133
Testicular self-examination, defined, 134, 179
Testicular torsion
 defined, 109, 134, 179
 symptoms, 134
 treatment, 135
Testis, undescended, defined, 132, 180
Testosterone
 deficiency
  defined, 53, 179
  diagnosis, 61
  replacement therapy, 62
 defined, 32, 179
 effects, 60
 effects in hormone replacement therapy, 48-49
 production decline, 60-61
 replacement therapy, 62
 role in male reproductive system, 60
Thioridazine, effects, 54
Thrombosis, birth control pill, 142
Thrush, defined, 116, 179
Thyroid problems, effects, 53
Tioconazole, effects, 119-120
Toilet paper, perfumed, effects, 118
Toys, sex, prevalence of use, 27
Tranquilizers, effects, 127
Transsexual, defined, 23, 179
Transvestism, defined, 23, 179
Trichomoniasis
 defined, 69, 78, 179
 diagnosis/treatment, 79
 prevalence, 69
 symptoms, 78-79
Tubal ligation, defined, 140, 180
TV, effects on sexual health, 11, 19-20

U

Ultrasound
 erectile dysfunction, 55
 infertilty, 161
 prostate cancer, 128
Uncircumcised, defined, 118, 180
Undescended testis, defined, 132, 180
Urethra, defined, 32, 180
Urethral suppositories
 costs, 57
 effects, 56, 57
Urethritis, defined, 122, 180
Urinary incontinence
 causes, 129
 defined, 129, 174
Urinary sphincter, defined, 126, 180
Urinary tract, defined, 45, 180
Urinary tract infection
 causes, 123
 defined, 43, 122, 180
 diagnosis/treatment, 124
 men, 124-125
 prevalence, 122
 risk factors, 123-124
 symptoms, 122
Uterus, defined, 35, 180
UTI. *See* Urinary tract infection

V

Vaccine, hepatitis, 94-95
Vacuum pump
  costs, 58
  effects, 56
  pros/cons, 58
Vagina, defined, 27, 180
Vaginal dryness
  causes, 43-44
  incidence, 46
Vaginal intercourse
  conception odds, 139
  positions, clitoral stimulation, 39
  risk levels, 104
Vaginal lips. *See* Labia majora; Labia minora
Vaginal pouch. *See* Condom, female
Vaginismus, defined, 44, 180
Vaginitis
  defined, 78, 109-110, 180
  symptoms, 78
Vaginosis. *See* Bacterial vaginosis
Vagistat-1, effects, 119-120
Valacyclovir, effects, 85, 86
Valtrex, effects, 85
Vas deferens, defined, 33, 180
Vascular surgery, effects, 56
Vasectomy, defined, 140, 181
Vasocongestion, defined, 31, 181
Venereal disease. *See* Sexually transmitted disease
Vesicle, defined, 82, 181
Viagra
  costs, 57
  effects, 56-57
Vibramycin, effects with chlamydia, 71-72
Vibrators
  defined, 27, 181
  drawbacks, 42
  effects, 41
  prevalence of use, 27
Viracept, effects, 99
Viramune, effects, 99
Vitamin C, effects, 89
Vulva, defined, 35, 181
Vulvar pruritis, defined, 118, 181
Vulvovaginal candidiasis. *See also* Yeast infection
  defined, 43, 181
VVC. *See* Vulvovaginal candidiasis

W

Warts, genital. *See also* HPV
  causes, 89
  diagnosis, 89
  forms, 89
  Pap smears, 91-92
  treatment, 89

Withdrawal
  defined, 141, 181
  effectiveness, 141
Women
  aging and sexuality, 44-49
  anorgasmia, 40-41
  contraceptives. *See also* Birth control pill; Cervical cap; Condom, female; Diaphragm; Fertility awareness method; Implants; Injectables; IUD; Rhythm method; Symptothermal method
    burden on women, 17
  ejaculation, 37
  excitement, physical changes, 35-38
  infertility, 161-162
  orgasm, 13, 14, 37-43
  reproductive system, anatomical illustration, 166
  reproductive tract disorders. *See* Bacterial vaginosis; Urinary tract infection; Yeast infection
  sex flush, 36
  sexual arousal, physical changes, 35-37
  STD, burden on women, 17

X

X-rays, erectile dysfunction, 55

Y

Yeast infection. *See also* Vulvovaginal candidiasis
  causes, 116-118
  defined, 43, 181
  HIV-related, 96
  long-term effects, 121
  pregnancy, 121
  prevalence, 117
  recurrent, 120
  symptoms, 118
  vs. bacterial vaginosis, 116
Yeast infections
  diagnosis, 119
  men, 118-119
Yocon. *See* Yohimbine
Yogurt, effects, 114
Yohimbine
  defined, 56, 181
  effects, 56, 59
Yohimex. *See* Yohimbine

Z

Zalcitabine, effects, 98
Zidovudine, effects, 98
Zithromax, effects, 71-72
Zoloft, effects, 50
Zovirax, effects, 85